30p

Travel
in
Retirement

Books by Dan Lees

FICTION

The Rainbow Conspiracy
Zodiac
Rape of a Quiet Town
Elizabeth R.I.P.
Our Man in Morton Episcopi
Mayhem in Morton Episcopi

NON FICTION

Beginner's Luck
The Champagne Fitness Book
Offbeat Somerset
Cooking in Retirement

Travel in Retirement

DAN & MOLLY LEES

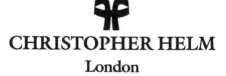

CHRISTOPHER HELM
London

© 1988 Dan and Molly Lees
Line illustrations by David Farris
Christopher Helm (Publishers) Ltd, Imperial House,
21-25 North Street, Bromley, Kent BR1 1SD

British Library Cataloguing in Publication Data

Lees, Dan
  Travel in retirement.
  1. Aged—Travel
  I. Title   II. Lees, Molly
  910′.2′02   G151
  ISBN 9-7470-2005-1

Typeset by Florencetype Ltd, Kewstoke, Avon
Printed and bound in Great Britain
by Billings and Sons Ltd, Worcester

Contents

Acknowledgements

We would like to thank the following people and organisations for their help in the preparation of this book: Philip Bradford, British Rail; British Waterways Board; The Caravan Club; Thomas Cook Ltd; Tony Court, AA Public Relations Officer, West & Wales Region; Melanie Crook; Ann Doolan; Paul Emery, Swift Travel; Tony Ferrand, editor Retirement World; John & Zena Gardner; Peter Gould, Regional Secretary, Ramblers Association; Alan Harrison, British Rail; Bill Ireson; Molly & David Jones; Patrick Leal; Hall Newell; Fred Peddle; Barbara Rees, Regional Director Age Concern; Ted & Dorothy Rogerson; The Royal Yachting Association; SAGA; Ken Smith, Roman City Holidays; Somerset & Avon Police, Crime Prevention Department; John Steed, Beacon Alarms; Thomson Young At Heart Holidays; T.P.S. Travel Press Services; Wessex Narrow Boats; Richard Wigmore.

1

Congratulations!
You Are Now an Aristocrat

For anyone who is working full-time, travel can be Hell, and it will come as no surprise to those who remember the horror of taking fractious children on high-season package tours to learn that the word travel orginally derived from the Latin word for torture.

Travel in retirement on the other hand is—or should be—a completely different experience, a leisurely and enjoyable progress, with the added bonus that, in most cases, those who are no longer working full-time pay only a fraction of what the same journey costs everyone else.

The secret is that, when it comes to travel, time really is money and retired people not only have time to spare but often, for the first time in their lives, are masters of it. This makes retirement the ideal time to travel and retired folk the aristocrats among travellers.

For most of us retirement is the first time that we have been able to travel for our own enjoyment without having to consider the exigencies of business, the demands of bosses, the tyranny of a holiday roster or the inflexible time-table imposed by school holidays. We are the masters now and that makes all the difference, but it is a heady freedom and a state of affairs which takes some getting used to.

I remember the days when I worked as a reporter for a national newspaper and there was always a race to get the story; we all drove like maniacs, taking the most horrifying risks in all sorts of weather. The point is that we were so conditioned to believe that speed was all-important that we took the same risks when covering a banal 'Silly Season' funny as we did when working on a potential front-page lead. Not only that, but the conditioning still held on our rare days off when our wives would be subjected to bad tempered cursing and hair-raising overtaking on what ought to have been carefree excursions and shopping trips. As far as I was concerned the conditioning even carried over for years after I had left the paper and it is only quite recently that my driving has become less frenetic—and a great deal

1

more enjoyable. Perhaps age has something to do with it but, nevertheless, I remember my older colleagues—especially the photographers who not only had to rush to the story but also had to get back quickly with their pictures—driving like madmen and having near heart attacks when they were held up in traffic jams.

The secret of enjoyable travel is being able to relax and at least those of us who are older and no longer working in accordance with someone else's time-table can learn how to take things easy. These days, whenever I'm tempted to rush myself into an ulcer, I think of the young bull and the old bull standing on a hilltop overlooking a lush valley in which a herd of sleek Jersey cows were grazing. 'Come on,' yelled the young bull excitedly, 'let's run down and make love to one of those beautiful cows.' The old bull replied contentedly, 'No, son. Let's amble down and make love to them all.'

Seriously though, the sooner we realise that no one is breathing down our necks anymore—and that even if boats, trains and planes won't wait for us we now have the time to catch them in comfort and if we miss them it's not the end of the world—the sooner we can begin to consider the other advantages of travel in retirement.

Before we start thinking about these in detail, however, it may be as well to point out that Molly and I regard as 'travel' any trip outside the home, whether it's a short walk or voyage round the world. We also believe that travel only broadens the mind if you are prepared to let it and that you can get more enjoyment out of a stroll in the country with your eyes open than a round the world cruise with them shut. As for retirement, we are using this to mean anyone who isn't working full-time for a boss or a business, whether they have taken early retirement at 45 or soldiered on to 65. Retirement can mean quitting work while still relatively young with a platinum handshake and a massive pension or finding yourself at 60 or 65 plus with nothing but the not over-generous State pension.

Obviously, there are differences between the travel requirements of the wealthier younger-retired and elderly pensioners but between the two extremes there are people who share a great deal of common ground while, when it comes to age, most of us with a bit of luck ought one day to qualify.

Money is one thing which worries many people on the verge of retiring; they feel they would like to travel but fear they won't be able to afford it. In fact most people find they are better off when they retire than they feared, mainly because their outgoings are considerably less than they've been for most of their working lives. People find, for example, that their houses are now paid for or, if they have moved to a smaller home, they have a useful capital sum in addition to having no mortgage to pay. Other expensive capital items like furniture, cars, domestic equipment and so on are usually paid for, commuter season

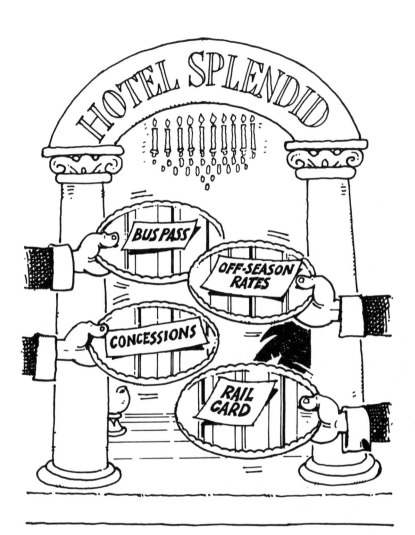

tickets are no longer a regular expense and retired people don't usually need to buy as many clothes as people who are working. In most cases, too, the children will have left home and, even if there are grand-children, spoiling a grandchild on occasions is nothing like the daily financial drain involved in bringing up one's own children.

3

Another important point is that once you retire, instead of having to find money for National Insurance, private insurances, pension schemes and the like, people usually start paying you—a double gain that can be very useful indeed.

Time not money is the deciding factor when it's a question of whether or not to travel. For example, although my parents were reasonably well-off—and my father was a railway executive who qualified for free travel facilities throughout most of Europe—they did considerably less travelling than Molly's parents who, as a retired couple with just a little more than the State pension, were able to spend six months out of every year travelling and living abroad. They travelled from one end of Europe to the other in huge elderly motor-cars, usually pulling equally elderly caravans and often finding themselves in some of the most expensive places in the world where they managed to live the life of Reilly on very little money. We learned a great deal about travel in retirement from Molly's mother and father, in fact it was they who introduced us to the French Riveria where we lived happily for several years in virtual semi-retirement, proving to our own satisfaction that you don't need a fortune to travel or live abroad.

Since returning to Britain I've done quite a lot of business travelling, most of which I found enjoyable, but it bears no relation whatsoever to any form of travel where you are spending your own money and taking your time. I've also done quite a lot of travel writing, which involves travelling under splendid conditions, most of which can be duplicated by retired people who, like travel writers, can make their journeys well outside peak season, have the time to organise their activities and are able to keep costs to themselves down to a minimum.

In this book there is a great deal about how retired people can save money and get the optimum value for the money they do spend. Sometimes our hints and tips about travelling will seem so simple and obvious as to be hardly worth mentioning. Common sense really, but they are things we had to learn the hard way so perhaps they are not all that common after all, and if a few of them are new to most people we'll be happy. Mainly, however, we'll be pounding away at the fact that, for retired people, time really is better than money—a near magic resource which can make travel not only cheaper but a lot more enjoyable and rewarding.

The reason we are so insistent about this is that work is habit forming and it's no use trying to kid ourselves that a lifetime of discipline at school and in the workplace hasn't had an effect on our lifestyle. Some people in fact find it very difficult to come to terms with retirement at all because they have been so conditioned by work that they feel lost and uncomfortable without a job to go to every day. This is where travel in retirement can become not merely enjoyable but an essential part of the retirement process, helping us to overcome what many feel to be a brutal change of routine, in the same way that a honeymoon helps single people make the adjustment to married life. At the other end of the scale are those people who seem content to spend all their waking hours in front of a television set and, while I often feel more kinship with them than with the workaholics, I have to admit that it's not all that life-enhancing or even healthy in the long run. Mind you, workaholics who decide to travel in their retirement can always make themselves masters of travel planning and tactics while those of us who prefer to read or watch TV can learn a lot from armchair travelling before tackling the real thing.

Travel has something for almost every retired person, providing as it does new goals to replace the career and business aims that once occupied so much of our time.

Planning for travel is fun, besides being important for older people who can use it to enable them to avoid many of the annoyances that the very young take in their stride. Kipping down on someone's hard floor, for example, may be fine for teenagers but, although once in a while it may be part of the adventure of travel at any age —as an Australian pensioner friend of ours discovered recently when he arrived unexpectedly and found all the beds in our house full—it's not something you want to do all the time once you hit 30, never mind 60.

One thing we can learn from today's young travellers is how to get about the world cheaply—and for that matter how to live cheaply practically anywhere—but it's as well to know exactly what you are letting yourself in for. As a young teenager, for example, our daughter absolutely revelled in a coach trip to Spain which Molly and I found only just bearable. Come to think of it, though, Molly's mother and aunt, who were both pushing 70, had no complaints, so it must have been because at that particular time we were too old to travel as relaxed teenagers and too young to take it as easy as travellers in retirement.

Travel in retirement can help to keep us physically fit and mentally alert, while spending a few weeks in the sunshine, away from the rigours of the British winter, can help us avoid strength-sapping coughs and colds as well as cutting down on fuel bills. Nowadays many holiday resorts run their own 'keep fit' programmes with carefully graded activities, walks and so on to suit all ages and we'll be looking at some of these in the context of retirement.

As I discovered while writing *Beginner's Luck*—in which I tried out 30 or so sports and pastimes—no matter where you go you'll find enthusiasts and experts who are only too anxious to welcome new-comers, whatever their age, either as participants or as helpers. This is an ideal way to make new friends, which of course is an important bonus for those of us who travel in retirement.

With a bit of luck we will all live long enough to become old people—as opposed to older people—but this is no reason not to continue to enjoy the benefits of travel. Even if we are handicapped—and age itself brings handicaps, if only a diminishing ability to hurl heavy luggage about—there are still plenty of ways to enjoy travel and to make things easier. They do require more planning but you have the time for that when you are retired. We have also discovered a special vacation project which provides a change of scene for people who need constant care of the type provided in nursing homes.

Meanwhile for those of us who are still reasonably fit, travel in retirement is a question of deciding what sort of travel we want to undertake, assessing our physical and financial capabilities and being prepared to take advantage of what is, in essence, a very privileged position. As we shall see, the privileges depend on our having time available for travel when most people are too busy or can't get time off work at a day's notice. This makes us Very Important Passengers on buses, coaches, trains, ships and aeroplanes, as we are able to fill seats and hotel rooms that would otherwise remain empty.

We'll be looking at a great many travel bargains offered to older people by all sorts of companies and we think it's important to bear in mind that there is no suggestion of charity involved, no question that the firms concerned are doing us a favour or taking pity on our advanced years. The fact is that we are the only people who can prevent their businesses from being unbalanced by high-season feasts and low-season famines and this is why they offer us such splendid deals. That being said, it is up to us to strike the best bargains we can, while emphasising that we are not second-class citizens of the travel world but valued clients entitled to the best that can be provided for our money. In fact, as I suggested earlier, we are the aristocrats of travellers, mainly because as retired folk we are in a position to travel in a way once enjoyed only by aristocrats with private means and no occupation.

There was a time when only aristocrats travelled for pleasure—while journeymen, soldiers, pedlars and the like travelled because they had to—and it's perhaps worthwhile to compare their situation to ours. First and foremost aristocrats, having by and large no need to earn a living, had time at their disposal, which meant they had no need to hurry and were able to travel as and when they wished. They had time to plan and prepare their journeys with care in order to maximise their comfort and to make sure that they arrived at their destinations refreshed rather than jaded. Having no time-table to which they were forced to adhere, they were usually unworried about delays and were happy to accept drinks, meals and so on proffered by way of compensation with good grace.

There were other ways in which aristocrats made travel easy for themselves, one of which was to maintain first-class contacts with their friends and relations, wherever they might be, a valuable but time-consuming exercise which can only be fully exploited by ladies and gentlemen of leisure—which is what most of us become as soon as we pick up our golden handshake, our long-service watch or our redundancy notice and join the ranks of the retired.

We'll be looking at the advantages of building up a travel in retirement network of useful addresses and passing on some of the things we have learned about 'guestmanship' but, although the savings involved can be considerable and, for retired people, extremely important, they are not really half as important as the new friends that can be made and the old friendships that may be rediscovered.

In much the same way we shall be suggesting ways in which it is possible to travel cheaply, to live in the sun for a modest expenditure and to find entertainment for next to nothing in most places. Here again, the savings are important (and we hope that anyone who reads this book will save its cost many times over) but we are much more concerned that those people who decide to travel in retirement, whether their journeys are long or short, staid or adventurous, modestly priced or costly, should enrich the quality of their lives and make retirement the joyous time it should be.

2

Walking on the Bright Side

There's an old Chinese saying to the effect that 'a journey of a thousand miles begins with a single step' and, while it applies to everyone, this particular piece of folk wisdom is extremely appropriate for those of us who have reached retiring age or are close to it.

Of course not everyone is as lazy as I am but I must confess that these days I find it takes an effort just to get out of my comfortable armchair, never mind begin a journey of a thousand miles. Until recently it was Molly who was the real walker in our family. Her parents loved walking—real walking that is, not dawdling arm-in-arm behind leashed-in children—and as soon as her little legs could carry here she was accompanying them on hikes across vast tracts of Lancashire moorland to places like Rivington Pike and Owd Betts.

Throughout the early years of our marriage the mere mention of the word 'walking' produced a flood of stories of her precocious pedestrian feats—the implication being that if I would only get off my bottom we could share the joys of long country walks. She didn't succeed of course, mainly because I had usually been working hard and wanted nothing more than to curl up with a good book and a couple of bottles of beer.

Then overnight everything changed when I gave up my staff job and we went to live in the South of France, which was splendid fun but not the greatest career move I have ever made. Moneywise, our years in France were precarious, to say the least, and we never felt quite able to risk buying a car to replace the one we had sold to help finance the trip. With less money—and more time—at our disposal, we were in a position very similar to that of an officially 'retired' couple and it was then that we rediscovered our feet.

To my astonishment—and Molly's 'I told you so' glee—we found that walking, even in semi-retirement, was a rewarding exercise—and not merely financially. For me it was a new experience to walk even as far as the market and it wasn't long before I discovered that it's also

8

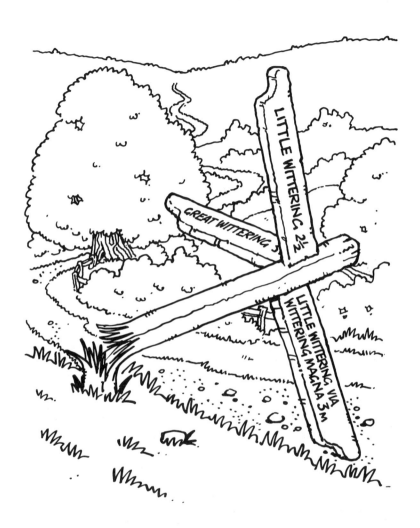

A good map is essential . . .

a great way to meet people and that an excursion to the shops can often take most of the morning.

In France we found ourselves walking the hills of the 'back country' for pleasure and even walking fairly long distances for interviews—which surprised people like Harold Robbins. He took pity on us and had us driven home in a Cadillac.

9

Knowing that walking was possible—this is by no means as silly as it sounds—proved useful when we came back to England jobless and broke. We moved in with Molly's parents and, as an interim measure, I took a 'must have a car' selling job at which I was quite successful—on foot.

An Australian friend of ours, Hal Newell—an experienced solo world traveller—does a lot of walking between bus, train and boat trips, partly to save money and partly because he finds it the best way to see places and to get to know people. Walking is cheap and that's a real attraction for those of us who are travelling in retirement but, like most other things, it isn't totally free and there are one or two items on which it doesn't pay to economise.

It sounds trite but the first thing we should think about if we are going to do any walking at all is our feet. No kidding, unless feet go wrong they tend to get neglected, perhaps because they are furthest away from the command centre. Then again, if you are like me and tend to put on weight, the little devils become more difficult to reach as one gets older. Even if we are only using our feet to get around the house and to go shopping it is vital to keep them well looked after and it's worth while, if you have a memory like mine, to note down a regular foot-care session in your diary. If you intend doing more serious walking and suspect you might have trouble with your feet you could see your doctor or chiropodist, but if your feet are normally sound then reasonable care and good footwear, coupled with the retired traveller's take-it-easy approach should be sufficient.

For ordinary walking—shopping, walking round town and even short country walks on roads and decent paths—stout comfortable shoes will usually be all that's needed. For serious walking—which in my case is anything over 5 miles—a pair of walking boots is a good investment and these could cost anything from about £30 upwards. Of course they are meant to last and you should get a lot of mileage out of them. Make sure they are comfortable to start with and do run them in by wearing them in the garden and round the house and then for short walks before giving them a road test over longer distances.

Lightweight boots are a good choice for all-the-year-round walking but they can cost more than £40 a pair so, unless you have decided that you want to do a lot of walking, it could be best to begin with the most comfortable suitable footwear you already possess. In fact the same thing applies to a lot of walking equipment and most people already have some sort of rainwear they can use when they start walking. For instance, I'm very fond of my cagoule which rolls up small enough to go in the pocket of my zip-up heavy cotton jacket which will also take waterproof trousers, sandwiches and maps so I can happily walk for a whole day without having to carry anything—

or even longer if I can drip-dry my shirt, socks and underpants overnight.

Walking is an ideal means of travelling in retirement, especially as it helps keep you fit without too much exertion. It may even help you live longer—the Secretary of the Ramblers Association, Tom Stevenson, lived to be 94 and one middle-aged walking enthusiast friend of ours claims that he is rapidly becoming used to people whistling past him on hills and stopping at the top to say to him things like 'I'm having my seventy-eighth birthday next week.'

Making a Start

If you haven't done any walking at all then begin by walking to the shops or to church or the pub, extending the distance until you can do 2 or 3 miles with comfort. Take it easy, rest when you want to and don't carry too much shopping. Get used to looking—really looking—at your surroundings and if you meet someone who wants to chat, stop and talk.

I find that in towns, especially in the older parts, you miss a great deal if you don't look up occasionally to check out the facades, the decorative windows, gargoyles and so on. Mind you, it pays to be careful of traffic and—unless you are a practical joker like my grandfather—to move on before you collect a crowd. A small notebook or sketchbook and pencil are useful for these trips and for later reference when you are trying to remember where on earth you have seen a similar doorway or chimney stack. You could find yourself becoming quite knowledgeable about local architecture.

Guided Walks

Most towns and cities run guided tours and you can find out about these from the Tourist Information Centre or the local library. Such tours make an enjoyable outing and are a splendid way of making new friends, as well as being an easy introduction to longer walks. Tour guides—often retired folk themselves—are usually extremely considerate and will match the pace of the slowest member of their party. However, if you are severely handicapped, it is worthwhile enquiring if there are any special arrangements for people with mobility problems.

Incidentally, Molly and I like to go on conducted walks wherever possible when we visit a new town; it may seem a bit 'touristy' but it adds to your enjoyment of the place if you know a bit about its history and its most interesting buildings. You can always strike out on your own later and, if you decide to stay in a place, put together 'personal' walks to suit the tastes of family and friends when they visit you. We started doing this when we lived in France and continued with it in Bristol and the West Country where Molly can quickly work out a Georgian Tour, a Medieval Tour, an Ancient Churches Tour and so on while I am happy to take visitors on my Historic Pubs Tour.

Rambling

After a bit of modest walking of this sort you should be ready for the big time—but do take it easy. A good plan is to join your local Ramblers Association (RA), membership of which ranges from teenagers to nonagenarians so you should find quite a few retired folk to keep you company. There are a lot of advantages to walking with others—about 20 people in one party is usual—one of which is that you will be with experienced walkers who will give you all the practical advice you need and make sure you don't overtax yourself. Peter Gould, a Regional Secretary of the Ramblers Association explained, 'No one is out to break records so the pace is geared to that of the slowest members of the group. We are walking for fun and we want people to enjoy themselves.'

The official ruling of the Ramblers Association regarding new-comers is that 'inexperienced ramblers should not be expected to walk more than 8 miles in a full day or 5 miles in half a day' and many local groups have evening walks of only 4 miles which are an excellent way of starting. Peter's group, for instance, go on 4 mile Thursday walks and usually stop for a break halfway round at a convenient pub.

The style of the walks themselves depends on the character and inclination of the group leader and while some like to get on with the walk others like to stop and look at every butterfly. The main thing is that, as Peter Gould emphasises, 'everyone is walking for pleasure which makes it ideal for retired people' and after the first few forays you should be reasonably clear whether or not you will be able to take part in normal rambling activity without holding people back.

Across gently undulating countryside 10 to 15 miles a day is a reasonable distance for experienced ramblers, although terrain and weather conditions will affect your speed; obviously you won't be expected to walk as fast over hilly ground as on the flat, and muddy conditions will slow you down as well. Hills are taken into account when walks are planned and, as a rule, each 1,000 feet of ascent or descent reduces the ramblers' norm by between 1 and 2 miles. For walks outside the group's immediate area, transport—perhaps by hired coach or minibus—is often arranged, so don't be put off joining a group if you don't have a car.

Once you have had some experience of walking with a group you may well wish to try walking on your own or with a friend or partner—in which case it makes sense to tell some responsible person where you are going and what time you expect to be back. You may have noticed that many ex-soldiers announce—often rather rudely— that they are going to attend to a call of Nature, because they became used to warning their mates that they were going where there might be danger, and while you don't have to take things quite that far it's a good idea to get into the habit of telling someone where you are off to.

Walking in Britain

In Britain—unlike many other countries—you can walk, away from the traffic, on paths running through farmland or on uncultivated hills and mountains. There are also many splendid long-distance routes. In England and Wales there are more than 100,000 miles of public footpaths and bridleways and walkers have the right to use any of them.

There are also a large number of public paths in Scotland but nobody knows just how many because they are not recorded and mapped as they are in England. As a rule of thumb, large gentlemen with pronounced Scottish accents wearing Harris tweed plus-fours and carrying shot guns should be regarded as knowing precisely where the paths are. Many of them will turn out to be helpful once they are convinced that you really are out for a walk and are not after game.

Many paths are now signposted where they join metalled roads and a small but growing number are marked with yellow or blue arrows so that you can be sure you are keeping to the right of way. You will find, however, that in some places the path has been ploughed over and crops planted in it—which is illegal. You are entitled to walk through the crop, sticking as close as is practicable to the line of the path, but, being a considerate person or a coward—I'm never quite sure which—I usually look for a way round.

It's a good idea to have a decent map and, where possible, a *Path Guidebook* with you—especially for the tricky places where the path goes across a farmyard or through someone's garden—and if there's anyone around it's always pleasanter to ask permission, even though you are sure you have right on your side. That way you are more likely to be warned if your legal right of way is being temporarily impeded by large and unfriendly animals.

Britain offers a wide range of scenery from the mountainous areas of the Scottish Highlands, the Welsh Border and the English Lake District to the gentler countryside of the Cotswolds, the Chilterns and the North and South Downs. You can walk along Offa's Dyke—the great earthwork built about AD 800 to mark the frontier between Mercia and Wales; Hadrian's Wall, built by the Romans as a defence against marauding tribesmen from the north; or the ancient trackways along the chalk hills of the south—the prehistoric trade routes and the 'herepaths' or warpaths of the Saxon armies.

It pays to be careful though; last time I was walking along the marvellous Ridgeway close to Avebury I turned round to urge the distaff side of the family to get a move on, twisted my foot and was unable to walk for days.

Long-Distance Paths

One advantage of walking in retirement is that you now have time to walk fairly long distances while taking things easy in terms of daily mileage. With no job to rush back to you can pace yourself comfortably and take days off in between if you feel like it. You'd probably need well over a month, for example, to cover the 250 miles of the Pennine Way—a walk which Molly, as a true Lancashire lass, insists we must try one day soon.

Careful preparation and planning are essential for long-distance walks and as well as arranging accommodation along the way and kitting yourself out in comfortable clothes you must be able to cope with rapid changes in weather. A small backpack with wide padded straps is probably the best way of toting anything you need *en route* but the most important thing is not to overestimate the distance you can travel each day, particularly in the early stages.

Of course you don't have to tackle the whole of any of the routes but it's worth knowing that as well as the Pennine Way there are:

The Cleveland Way	93 miles	North-east England
Offa's Dyke Path	168 miles	English/Welsh Border
Pembrokeshire Coast Path	167 miles	South-west England
Ridgeway Path (ouch!)	85 miles	Central Southern England
South Downs Way	80 miles	South-east England
North Downs Way	141 miles	South-east England
Wolds Way	79 miles	North-east England
South-west Way	515 miles	Coast of South-west England

The South-west Way sounds pretty daunting but it is more feasible for retired people than for those in full-time employment. One Londoner I heard of, who had never walked much further than to his local pub before, just took off with only a rather objectionable dog for

14

company—he was supposed to be minding it for his sister—and walked the entire distance. But, on the whole, and especially for older people, it's essential to have put in some good walking practice before tackling a long path. However, the South-west Way really is a splendid walk, not to mention a considerable achievement, and Molly and I are looking forward to doing it although she insists we walk the Pennine Way first.

The Ramblers Association can provide full details of all the official Long-Distance Paths, together with information about other long-distance routes devised by their members from existing path networks. Take advantage of their expertise and ask their advice at the planning stage.

As well as the official 'paths' there are plenty of places in Britain where walkers can roam over uncultivated countryside and these include 'access land' where formal agreements have been made—such as the 70 square miles of the Peak District National Park.

In England and Wales there is also Common Land—some 1,500,000 acres of it—which is privately owned but over which the local villagers enjoy grazing rights. The landowner is not allowed to enclose such lands and the public is usually free to wander over them at will, although strictly speaking they have no legal right to do so. There are some huge areas of the Pennines, the moorlands of Dartmoor and the fells of the Lake District which have this sort of status but, as I know from both personal experience and from having worked on 'lost hiker' stories for newspapers, these are places which need to be treated with respect. Even in midsummer the weather can change dramatically so do let people know your route and what time you expect to arrive at your next port of call and, above all, take the experts' advice. If the locals advise against tackling the next stretch that day you are better off exploring the village and trying out the local hostelries. If you've booked in at other places along your route, however, don't forget to let them know that you are held up. They will appreciate it and so will the Rescue Services who might otherwise think you are lost.

The same thing applies to those large areas of Scotland, especially in the Highlands, which are available to the walker. Take care at all times and if you plan to walk in the uplands between 1 July and 20 October make enquiries before setting out because it's the deer shooting season and some areas are closed to walkers.

National Parks

In Britain the National Parks are not owned by the State and much of the land is in private hands, which means that you have to keep to the paths and public areas. In practice this is nothing like as restrictive as it sounds and most of the legislation, as in the case of what are called Areas of Outstanding Natural Beauty (AONB), is aimed at making sure that these places remain unspoiled by over-enthusiastic entrepreneurs.

The Country Code

Mind you, it's not just the builders and developers who are capable of spoiling the countryside for others and while we mature people are better behaved than most—naturally—it's worth taking a look at the Country Code which is largely common sense and of course applies to everyone, whatever their means of locomotion.

Enjoy the countryside and respect its life and work
Guard against all risk of fire
Fasten all gates
Keep your dogs under close control
Keep to public paths across farmland
Use gates and stiles to cross hedges, fences and walls
Leave livestock, crops and machinery alone
Take your litter home
Help to keep all water clean
Protect wildlife, plants and trees
Take special care on country roads
Make no unnecessary noise

Where to Stay

Being retired brings many advantages when it comes to accommodation, both when you are travelling and when you reach your destination.

Travelling at off-peak times, for example, means that you should benefit from off-season rates, special offers and so on and it is as well to remember that as a retired person you've time to ask about special rates—and you should.

Most hotels and guest houses have rooms which are standing empty during the off season and this makes the owners cry a lot. In order to fill these empty rooms many advertise special rates—'away breaks' and so on—and it's always worthwhile when making preliminary enquiries to ask if the particular establishment offers reduced rates for older people. Local Tourist Boards can be helpful with accommodation lists—it's best to give them some idea of your price range—and organisations like the Automobile Association (AA) produce excellent guides to guest houses and inns as well as hotels. You can ask your local library to look out appropriate publications for you, especially if they have a reference section.

How Retirement Can Mean Instant Rejuvenation

It comes as a pleasant surprise to many retired people to learn that, when it comes to travel, for a small sum they can recover their lost youth. All you have to do is to join the Youth Hostels Association (YHA). Membership is open to anyone over the age of 5; there's absolutely no upper age limit and the only snag is that, being over 21, you'll have to pay £6 to join—which even so is far from excessive. The YHA has 260 hostels, not only in the National Parks and on the long-distance paths but in cities, towns and at the seaside as well.

If you are using a hostel for the first time it's not a bad idea to try a 'superior' one first as this will enable you to find out whether hostelling is for you. You can test the water for a couple of nights by paying a guest subscription and, while you'll be paying the senior nightly rate, as this is unlikely to be more than £4 per person for a hostel graded 'superior' it is still a bargain. The 'special' class is more like a hotel while the 'simple' grade means just that. The 'standard' grade hostels have a WC for every ten beds, a washbasin for every six and there is hot and cold water, often with showers as well. There are cooking facilities, some form of heating in the common, quiet and dining rooms, a small store and a resident warden. Any retired person who has served in the forces will find standard grade hostels more than acceptable, but have a trial run before embarking on a hostelling marathon—just in case.

Hostels are available for members who travel by car or bicycle as well but they are often sited in places which make them particularly suitable for walkers. One of the most spectacular is the newest, called simply The Ridgeway, near Wantage, built on the site of an old chalk quarry halfway along the Ridgeway, high up on the Berkshire Downs, with superb views over the Vale of the White Horse. There are four bunk cabins, excellent facilities and even an outdoor swimming pool.

Specialist magazines, such as *Country Walking*, are a good source of information about accommodation with a surprising number of farms and small guest houses offering bed and breakfast for as little as £10 a night and even less out of season.

Walking Abroad

Unlike Britain, walking in many other countries is largely restricted to the relatively few long-distance paths—like the *sentiers de grande randonnée* in France—and off-road walking may well be frowned upon. In some ways this tends to be restrictive, but in most countries the side roads and by-ways make for enjoyable walking and official walking routes, such as those in Germany and Austria, have long been recognised as tourist attractions which usually means that they are well maintained and signposted. In Austria, for example, they are often an off-season alternative to ski-ing and for this reason are well supplied with cafes and restaurants. The Austrian Tyrol in particular is one of my favourite places for cheap early summer walking, using off-season packages from as little as £59 a week including travel, accommodation and food. Most of the vast ski-holiday infrastructure is available to you which means that you can whistle up mountains in comfortable ski-lifts and then start walking. The ski-lifts are still on the pricey side, though, even out of season, so it's reassuring to know that there are plenty of good walks much lower down, linking picturesque villages with friendly little inns and cafes.

If you have tried youth hostels in Britain and found you like them you will be pleased to know that there are some 5,000 of them in more than 50 countries from Argentina to Zimbabwe. All of them accept senior members with the notable exception of Bavaria, where for some reason the age limit is 27.

The standard of hostels in Europe ranges from excellent to just fair and as a rule of thumb the further north they are the more likely they are to match up with the British ones—or even beat them. One advantage of trying out a couple of hostels close to home before venturing abroad is that you will probably meet someone who knows the hostels in the part of the world you want to visit and who can 'mark your card'.

Travellers in retirement can save a small fortune by using the facilities offered by the YHA but there are other ways of seeing Europe on foot and it might be advisable to begin with an organised walking holiday.

One of Molly's aunts—in her mid-seventies—is an ardent hill walker and rambler and has had several walking trips abroad. So, if you are reasonably fit, age is no bar as there are special holidays for 'Senior Ramblers' in all parts of the world. (Holiday Fellowship is one of the better companies in this field and can be particularly recommended for women travelling on their own.) You could try, for instance, a trip to Saalbach to the south-west of Salzburg—a holiday village which makes a great walking centre, with cable-cars and chair-lifts to take you up to where the real scenery begins. This would cost you quite a bit in June or September for a fortnight's half pension at a family run hotel, and it is a bit pricey compared to the package trips, but the main advantage is that you have the choice of going off on your own, or in an informal group or with a group leader.

Ideally the way to begin walking in retirement, if you intend eventually to tackle long distances, would be to start rambling and hill walking with a local group, after which you could try walks with a partner and solo walks, perhaps taking advantage of YHA facilities.

You could then try a foreign walking holiday of the sort described above, perhaps following that with walking with a partner.

Incidentally, if you do find that walking is one of your favourite methods of getting about you could combine it with other forms of transport like Hal Newell and our other Australian 'back packer' friend Liz Coats, or make it part of a caravan tour—or even part of a 'Journey of a Lifetime' with a trip to, say, Kashmir. You can get a 17-day senior tour which includes in the price three days on a houseboat near the capital, three days in a mountain resort and six days on trek.

Once you've got the taste for walking, the world—as Hilda Ogden puts it—'is your lobster' and it could all start with nothing more adventurous than a stroll in the countryside.

Equipment

In summer, stout shoes will serve in most parts of Britain but if you are going into the hills you will need proper boots with 'Vibram' or 'Commando' soles. A windproof and if possible waterproof anorak is a must and, being something of a cissie, I like waterproof trousers as well.

You won't need a big rucksack to start with as all you'll need for a couple of hours walking will go into your pockets but when you do buy a backpack make sure it's comfortable and that you don't have to be a contortionist to get it on and off.

Always take a good Ordnance Survey map and a compass. One misty stretch of moorland looks very much like another and the compass could prove invaluable—provided of course that you know how to use one. Modern compasses with a built-in magnifying glass are particularly useful, especially for older folk. If you were not a Boy Scout or Girl Guide and find compass work difficult, it might pay to go on a course. The YHA run one—a weekend course in compass and map skills in conjunction with SEAL Guides at Edale in Yorkshire.

Strangely enough, travel is often one of the walker's biggest expenses, because once you have exhausted the possibilities of your own locality you will need transport to get where you want to walk. This is where a book on travel in retirement comes in handy.

Useful Addresses

Country Walking (Exmoor), Combe Lodge Hotel, Ilfracombe, Devon. Telephone (0271) 64518. Brochure available.

English Tourist Board, 4 Grosvenor Gardens, London SW1 0GY

European Rambling Association, Fulkerstrasse 70, D.7000, Stuttgart 1, West Germany

Friends of the Earth, 377 City Road, London EC1V 1NA

Holiday Fellowship, HF Holidays Limited, Department GRO 6, PO Box 31, Leicester LE2 2YE. Excellent walking holidays—welcomes single retired people

Pennine Outdoor, Hardknott, Holmbridge, Huddersfield, Yorkshire. Telephone (0484) 684302. Fabric and pattern stockists. Useful if you want to make your own walking and waterproof clothing

Ramblers' Association, 1–5 Wandsworth Road, London SW8 2XX. Telephone (01) 582 6878. Well worth joining—the experts on all aspects of rambling and invaluable for advice on walking tours, etc.

Ramblers' Holidays, 13 Long Croft House, Fretherne Road, Welwyn Garden City, Hertfordshire. Telephone (0707) 331133

Scottish Tourist Board, 5 Waverley Bridge, Edinburgh EH4 3UV

Wales Tourist Board, PO Box 151, WDO, Cardiff CF5 1XS

Walk West, Yonder Marsh Farm, Nr Honiton EX14 9A4. Telephone 0460 34484. Guided tours with Mike and Peggy Harding. Brochure available

Walkabout Country Holidays. Brochure available from (02606) 263

Youth Hostels Association, Trevelyan House, 8 St Stephen's Hill, St Albans AL1 2DY. Telephone (0727) 55215. A wide range of cheap accommodation and useful information on the countryside

Further Reading

Collins New Generation Guides, Collins, London. First-class pocket book series on birds, wild flowers, etc.

Country Walking. A bi-monthly magazine with articles on short- and long-distance walking, planning routes, expert advice on equipment, details of short rambles, addresses of accommodation for walkers, holidays, clubs, tours, etc. obtainable from newsagents

La Grande Randonnée. Series of maps and guides on French long-distance paths. Available from Macarta, 122 Kings Cross Road, London

The Great Walking Adventure, Hamish Brown, Oxford Illustrated Press, Oxford. Humour, personal anecdotes and lots of useful information on tramping in places as far apart as Manchester and Marrakesh

The Long Distance Walker's Handbook, Barbara Blatchford, A&C Black, London. An invaluable guide to over 200 long-distance routes in Britain, ranging from 20 to 500 miles. Details are given of each route, with maps and relevant information

Ordnance Survey Maps. The 1:50,000 is most useful and can be obtained from good bookshops and main Post Offices. A must for all walkers

Rambler. A monthly magazine crammed with articles, members' experiences, advice from experts, latest in equipment, addresses for guided tours, etc.

Published by the Ramblers' Association (address above) and free to members

Ramblers' Yearbook. Annual, with full details of accommodation for walkers. Published by the Ramblers' Association (address above) and free to members

Walking in Britain. A (free) leaflet, excellent advice. Obtainable from Youth Hostels Association (address above)

YHA Guide. Annual, with details of all YHA hostels. Published by the Youth Hostels Association (address above)

3

Mister Peddle the Cyclist

Meeting Mr Peddle the Cyclist while researching a chapter on bicycles was like meeting Mr Bun the Baker while writing the history of bread making.

Certainly I found it difficult to believe my good fortune when I learned that Fred Peddle, in addition to being a former Council member of the Cyclists Touring Club (CTC), was 61-years-old and genuinely cycling in retirement.

Fred has been cycling since the early days of the Second World War, joined the CTC in 1943 and has been a keen cyclist ever since. He remembers paying £1 for his first bike, a secondhand model—which is just twice the price I paid for mine, a rugged affair held together largely by some twelve coats of lumpy black paint. I was very proud of it until my best friends—two brothers whose father managed a large department store—acquired spanking new Raleigh tourers with caliper brakes and three-speed gears.

Talking to Fred brought back all the anguish of seeing my proud steed reduced to the status of a pack mule among thoroughbreds but it also reminded me of the difficulty I had faced when learning to ride my first Fairy Cycle. I remembered too being quite upset because my cousin Valerie—a mere girl, if two years older—was able to ride rings round me on her own two wheeler.

Of course pushy cousins are unlikely to be a problem for older people learning to ride a bike for the first time and they won't have to risk grazed knees and the rest out of infantile macho pride. But could learning at retirement age be a problem? Said Fred, 'It depends on the individual; if they have a reasonable sense of balance there should be no difficulty, though some people will take longer to learn than others. Beginners should get a cyclist to help them—they've no need to be very experienced as long as they have the patience to walk along holding the saddle until the learner feels confident enough to have them let go.'

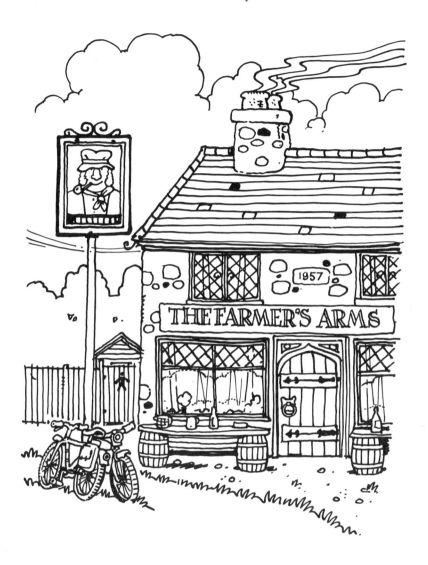

Fortunately for those of us who learned as children, the old saw about never forgetting how to swim or ride a bike really does hold good for cycling, although as Fred pointed out some people may find themselves wobbling a bit at first if they haven't been on a bike for decades. Learning to ride one is well worth the effort. Said Fred, 'It's a great thing for people to take up in their retirement, especially if they have another interest which can be enjoyed along with cycling. There are so many places to visit on short tours or on a day's ride and almost always cycling is the cheapest and best way to get to them.'

Fred uses his cycle for day-to-day transport and considers the cycle tracks in some towns and cities a boon for older cyclists as they keep them away from heavy traffic. 'The best time to learn – or to relearn – town riding,' he told me, 'is on Sunday morning when you can get used to the roads and road signs with nothing much to worry about in the way of traffic.'

Incidentally, I was interested to discover that the first brand-new bike I ever owned is still considered the best to learn on although the three-speed hub model now costs rather more than the £12 my father paid in 1939. However, you should still be able to get a decent secondhand example for around £60 – after which a lot depends on what you want to spend. Perhaps the best thing to do, after you have convinced yourself that you really can ride a bike, is to buy one of the cheaper 'company' lightweights made by a firm like Raleigh, which are excellent value and provide very good specifications at around £200.

A new touring model costs less at about £170 to £180 but they tend to be a bit on the heavy side and, as Fred put it, 'Anyone who wants to put in a genuine effort should go in for a lightweight. It's like fishing; you can fish with a bent pin and enjoy it but if you want to take up fishing there's a basic level of equipment you really need so you should buy the best you can afford.'

The good news for those of us who haven't cycled for a while or are still using old-fashioned machines is that in the last 40 years or so bicycles have improved almost as much as cars. You may not have the strength or the stamina you had when you were a kid but technology redresses the balance and the new lightweight multiple-geared machines are a joy to ride. I can vouch for this because quite recently I tried out a state of the art 'Mountain Bike' and found it tremendous fun; I was able to ride up and down rocky pathways which, even as a youngster, I would have found it hard to tackle on my old-style bike, even standing on the pedals.

One way of finding out if you are going to enjoy taking up cycling – before you spend a lot of money – is to hire a decent bike. (This can be done for less than £5 per day in most areas. One enterprising agency has set up a bike-hire shop at each end of the Bristol to Bath cycle track, so find out if in your area similar initiatives are being taken.)

Real cycling enthusiasts hate to be parted from their own machines even if they are travelling to the other side of the world, but for older people who prefer tootling to the Tour de France there are bikes for hire almost everywhere and they provide a splendid way of seeing a foreign country without the expense of hiring a car. Make sure you know the local ground rules; Holland, Belgium and many other countries have miles of first-class cycle paths on their roads but it's as well to check with the experts about different laws. The French, for instance, are no longer quite so insistent on their *priorité à droite* as they once were but you still have to watch out for the idiot who thinks that being on the right entitles him to come out of his driveway at sixty without warning.

In Britain it's essential to know the Highway Code as you not only need to know what you should do but what the vehicles sharing the road with you are likely to do. Our friend Ted Rogerson, who featured in our book *Cooking in Retirement*, cycled to work for years and after his retirement carried on cycling to and from his allotment. Like many other elderly cyclists he didn't bother about insurance because in his day it was far from usual but today it is absolutely essential, especially for older cyclists. Under current rules, had Ted been involved in an accident, he could have found himself lumbered with 10 per cent of any claim, even if the blame attached to him was minimal and 10 per cent of even a minor shunt with, say, a Jaguar or a Rolls would have made a shocking dent in his pension.

Fred Peddle mentioned the best way to go about it. 'You have to consider Third Party Insurance which is why it pays to join a club.' he said. 'The Cyclists Touring Club and the British Cycling Federation run schemes which insure their members. Membership of the CTC costs £15 for an adult but many retired people will find it even cheaper as there is a reduction for pensioners.'

Interestingly, about a quarter of the 40,000 plus CTC members are over 50 so there's no need to worry about being the only older person in the group. In fact, for retired people the club brings the added advantage of a chance to make new friends and the 54 district associations have an active social life. There is also a scheme under which you can advertise free of charge in the club's information-packed publications for a cycling companion—I'm told this not only works well but has even led to several romances. You'll also find details of touring and fixed-centre cycling holidays, many of which specifically state that they are suitable 'for all ages', are 'leisurely paced' and welcome 'potterers'.

Learning to Cycle

There's a world of difference between learning to ride a bike and learning cycling and Fred Peddle claims to be envious of people who are learning cycling today.

'I've seen people who came into cycling a few years ago and who were able to do things in weeks that it took me years to pick up.'

'But—what's to learn?' I asked. 'Once you can stay on the bike and know the rules of the road, isn't that all you need?'

Fred looked at me pityingly. 'What you learn is how to get the best out of cycling—you learn how to pace yourself and to know what you can do in a day, which is very important for older cyclists. You also learn how to incorporate special interests like archaeology, painting and so on into your cycling excursions.'

'Retired people have a definite advantage when it comes to planning because they have time and patience. It's very important, for instance, to make sure you have decent maps and good up to date guide books for the districts you visit. You can then check out the opportunities for, say, photography and be reasonably certain in advance that you know where you are going to find something to eat.'

'One thing you learn is just how versatile a machine the bicycle is. You can ride it, wheel it, lift it, carry it and—within reason—dump it while you go off on foot or some other form of transport.' This versatility makes it easier to follow a precept which Fred regards as one of the cardinal rules of modern cycling, especially for older people—namely, never to travel on main roads. It's dangerous and noisy and, besides, all the places you want to see are off the beaten track, which is usually why they have survived in the first place. Retired people can very quickly learn to seek out the cycle paths, lanes and by-ways and to plan their travelling to miss traffic where there is any. They are wise enough to know when to lie up for an hour if traffic is heavy or to take advantage of lunch time to get through somewhere like the Wye Valley while everyone else has stopped for a picnic.'

One thing all cyclists have to learn from experience is how to keep the rhythm going once they have established a comfortable pedalling, as opposed to road, speed—which means using the gears properly. Said Fred, 'Gears should be low. It's not so much that you can ride up the steepest hill but with proper gearing you can still keep going up a slope, whereas if you had to walk up it would take you far too long.'

Learning City Riding

There is no easy answer to the problems of city traffic and although experience helps it can be tricky. Roundabouts are one of the biggest hazards and sometimes, for older people especially, it is better to get off and walk. Juggernauts, too, are a hazard as they create a vacuum which tends to suck you in, especially when it's wet.

However, retired people—unlike workers—can avoid traffic by timing their trip and by planning crafty vehicle-free routes. Unlike motorists you can cross parks, cut through narrow passages and use side streets and footbridges. You can cycle round the back of main roads and even walk a bit here and there. It's a question of pitting your wits against the traffic and older people are usually better at this than the youngsters.

Touring in Britain

Touring in Britain—and elsewhere for that matter—is also a question of avoiding the traffic, much as in town riding, except that the planning is on a larger scale. Cyclists—even if they have to get off and walk—can use stepping stones, footbridges, paths with stiles and so on that are completely impassable for cars, a fact which sometimes provides miles of pleasurable traffic-free cycling.

When planning a route, make inquiries about any cycle paths in the area as new cycle ways are now being made fairly quickly. For example, it will soon be possible to ride on the Thames Cycle Way from the Cotswolds to Tower Bridge without seeing a car.

If you are lucky enough to have good cycling country close at hand you will have no trouble planning day trips but, once you have exhausted the local possibilities, you may wish to travel further afield—either to explore on your own or to take part in a group tour—without having to face a hard slog to a new centre.

It's Quicker by Rail

You could find that putting your bike—and yourself of course—on the train is the answer and, while we shall be examining the whole question of train travel in Chapter 8 it's worth mentioning that bikes travel free on all but 125 InterCity trains.

For retired cyclists this kind of charge is exactly the sort of challenge they enjoy and it's usually possible to find a non-125 service—some lines in fact are very good, the Cardiff to Portsmouth and the Cardiff-Crewe-Shrewsbury being two examples.

Retired people over 60 will almost certainly have invested in a Senior Citizen Rail Card which gives about one third off the price anyway, which means that if you take a regional, as opposed to a national Rover Ticket, you can use, say, the Wessex Card which would enable you to take your bike on the train free anywhere in the Bristol-Portsmouth-Weymouth triangle for the whole seven days. You could pop over to the Isle of Wight from Portsmouth and—staying at youth hostels—a week's combined cycle and rail touring would cost you only around £20—a good example of what travel planning in retirement can achieve. If you want to spend a little more money on your accommodation, local tourist offices will usually be able to help with lists—it's as well to let them know your price range—and you'll find lots of useful addresses in *Cycletouring*, the magazine of the CTC.

As Fred puts it, 'If only all older people would see the possibilities which are open to them instead of looking at their limitations they would get a great deal more out of their cycling—and out of their retirement.'

—or by Car

For older people, especially, the combination of bikes with other forms of transport is splendid and Molly and I consider that a car, a caravan and a couple of bicycles is just about the ideal arrangement.

One retired couple who opted for a car and cycles are Kate and Doug Jackman who took up cycling again after 30 years of motorised transport. Doug was the first to buy a bike, after his son pointed out 'the bargain of a lifetime' in one of his cycling mgazines, but it wasn't long before Kate too decided she could get a bit of exercise in her retirement by riding to the village. She acquired a folding bike that fitted into the back of the car, aiming to get more fun out of their longer trips. But Kate soon discovered that cycling in 1984—when she started again—wasn't anything like the cycling she remembered. 'The traffic was terrible and all the little hills seemed enormous.' Fortunately, she lives close to a cycle track and was able to get in some practice away from traffic and with no hills to worry about.

Doug's bike and the 'folder' packed into the family car but it soon became obvious that the folding cycle wasn't at its best on gradients so Kate changed to a ten-speed 'proper' bike; four months after taking up cycling again she and Doug had 'His' and 'Her' lightweight tourers carried on the car in a specially adapted roof rack. Doug and Kate are fairly typical of people who take up cycling after a lay off of several decades and their experience shows that it is quite feasible to become competent cyclists in retirement. They live in an area where there are plenty of varied day trips within a 25 mile drive including a run to the Wiltshire Cycle Track, part of which goes through the Longleat Estate. Their advice is always to have a particular destination in mind when setting out on a car-bike day excursion and always carry a good map of the area—like the relevant 1:50,000 Ordnance Survey sheet.

It's good to know that this combination of car and cycle travel is so enjoyable—even if Fred Peddle feels a little envious of people like the Jackmans who acquired a Claud Butler Majestic apiece after only four months of retirement cycling.

Cycling in Europe

Touring on the Continent is relatively easy—in fact in many ways it's easier to get to Europe from the south of England than it is to get up to the north of Scotland. The main difference is that England and

Wales have everything in the way of scenery and places to visit in a comparatively small compass whereas in Europe the interesting places are further apart. This makes combined train and cycle or car and cycle touring a very good bet. In most parts of Europe, quite apart from the Tour de France sort of cycling, people seem much more bicycle minded than in England. In France, for example, everyone seems to have a bike—often fitted with one of those tiny motors with the drive directly onto the front tyre. French motorists are used to coping with hordes of cyclists of all ages and while this doesn't make them any more courteous it does mean that they are skilled in avoiding two-wheeled machines—if only to save their paintwork.

Some of my most recent cycling in France was on the Riveria and although at first I used a bike because I couldn't afford a car I soon appreciated that in the high season a bicycle was quicker than a car. The doormen at many of the fancy Riveria hotels got quite used to my bike but some of the guests were astonished to see me arriving on it wearing evening dress and telling the doorman, '*Vous pouvez garer le Rolls.*'

To give you an idea of how you feel about touring abroad, without too much hassle, Brittany is a good place to start. There are plenty of organised low mileage tours and you will also get plenty of tips from the experts if you feel like venturing further afield.

World Cycling

Cyclists divide neatly into tootlers like ourselves, who use bikes as a cheap way of getting around with the added bonus of fresh air and exercise, and 'real' cyclists for whom cycling is a way of life. Mind you, joining a club can seriously endanger one's tootling status as you tend to be exposed to other people's enthusiasm, which could turn you into a real cyclist. This means, among other things, that if you go on a cycle tour in America or Tibet you will probably insist on taking your own machine with you. Fred Peddle—a real cyclist if ever there was one—told me, 'There's no difficulty whatsoever in taking bikes by air and if you are reasonably careful you can keep within the baggage allowance.'

This sounded a tall order but Fred took his bike to America for a tour of New England so he should know and, when you come to think of it, today's lightweight bikes weigh next to nothing when compared with the monster suitcases some people take on aircraft. 'Touring in that part of the world was great.' said Fred. 'We met a number of very friendly American cyclists too. It was an ideal way to see the country and there was plenty of reasonably priced accommodation.'

I'm not usually in favour of riding in great bunches but the best way to tackle foreign touring to the far-flung destinations now available is definitely on an organised tour like those run by the CTC—making sure of course that you are not going with a bunch of 25-year-old athletes. Once you have tried a foreign trip or two with a party you could try one on your own or with a companion.

Assisted Cycling

Apart from the tiny combustion engines already mentioned which, for some reason, have never caught on in Britain, there are now some useful electric motors which could well appeal to older riders.

The difference is that while combustion engines—even those driving direct on the wheel—are designed to be ridden under power most of the time and pedalled only when power is insufficient, the electrically-assisted bikes are meant to be pedalled most of the time with the electric motor being used mainly in emergencies. They are available both as 'do it yourself' conversions, with some motors having a range of about 15 miles, and as bikes with built in motors— with the same range. Some of the latter type use the three-speed hub as a gear box which makes them fairly sophisticated transport.

Cycles and Equipment

You can get some sort of boneshaker for under £50 but for a reliable secondhand machine a more realistic price would be about £70. At the other end of the scale you could easily pay well over £1,000 for a tailor-made lightweight and nearer £2,000 on the road for a bike with all the gubbins like lightweight paniers, trip computers and so on; one of our friends recently turned up with a bicycle for which he had paid more than we paid for our car!

However, unless you are rolling in cash, it's probably best to get on the road for less than £100 and then move up to more expensive gear later if you are getting a lot of use out of it. You could try a weekend at a centre which provides a comfortable base together with guidance on buying a bike, maintenance, route planning and so on. There, too, you should get the chance to try out different bikes such as tandems.

Clothing
You will need some sort of waterproof clothing and the choice lies between capes and suits. The traditional cape and sou'wester costs around £15 and Fred Peddle favours this rig because it protects both him and his bike and, he claims, doesn't funnel water into his shoes like waterproof trousers do.

Rainproof jackets and trousers can cost £100 or more but in my experience—and Fred's—are rarely totally waterproof. I used to favour a combination of cape, sou'wester and waterproof trousers—a belt and braces approach which kept me dry in anything bar a monsoon—but now that I can pick my times I'm beginning to think that a lightweight cape is quite enough to carry.

Lightweight comfortable shoes or trainers are fine for most cycling but high-tec has moved into this area and you can now buy special cycling shoes costing £50 and more.

Don't forget a light cotton hat in hot weather—it's easy to get the back of your neck sunburned even in Britain—and if you are good at sewing why not send for catalogues from one of the specialist fabrics firms who also stock patterns for outdoor gear suitable both for rambling and cycling.

Insurance

Insurance is a must these days and while you can insure privately it makes sense to join a club like the CTC because of the additional benefits. As well as free third party insurance, members get free legal aid, and advantageous terms when insuring their machine.

Clubs

As well as free insurance and so on, the CTC offers a full technical service, together with a touring service which will provide detailed routes for touring in Britain and a great deal of information about touring abroad. Members also receive a free handbook which includes lists of cycle repairers and so on and free copies of the club magazine *Cycletouring* which is published six times a year.

Cycling Checklist

This list is the absolute basic. Readers will probably want to add to it.
Waterproofs
Small repair kit (puncture repair kit, spare inner tube, tyre levers, 6 inch spanner and screwdriver
Waterproof saddlebag
Small pack of food and drink for emergencies
Oil and rag
Cycle lock and key

Useful Addresses

British Cycling Federation, 16 Upper Woburn Place, London WC1H 0QE. Telephone (01) 387 9320

Cyclecraft Holidays, 12 Morningside, Lancaster LA1 ASR. Holidays for those people wanting to try out bikes, learn about buying, maintaining and using them. Brochure available

Cyclists' Touring Club, 69 Meadrow, Godalming GU7 23HS. Telephone (04868) 7217. The experts—lots of benefits to members including insurance, advice, detailed routes, regular leaflets and magazines

Fellowship of Cycling Old Timers. Secretary/Treasurer: Jim Shaw, 2 Westwood Road, Marlow, Buckinghamshire. A club with many local branches for the older cyclist. Publishes a news magazine, holds meetings and outings, etc.

See Ireland by Bike, Enid House, Gunnersbury Lane, London

The Tandem Club, Box No TC1, c/o Cyclists' Touring Club (address above)

Tom Race, 22 Ringmore Rise, Forest Hill, London SE23 3DE. Hotel-based, leisurely-paced guided bicycle tours

Triskell Cycle Tours in Brittany, 35 Langland Drive, Northway, Sedley DY3 3TH. Telephone (09073) 78255. Brochure available

Further Reading

Bicycle Hire List. Obtainable from Cyclists' Touring Club (address above)

Bicycle Times. A monthly magazine. Cycling activities, rallies, maintenance tips, practical advice, readers' experiences, tandems. Obtainable from newsagents

Cycletouring. The magazine of the Cyclists' Touring Club. Free to members

Cycling World. A monthly newspaper with the latest on new machines, travel, rallies, holidays, etc. Obtainable from newsagents

England by Bicycle, Frederick Alderson, Star Books, London. A delightful, very readable account of one month's cycle tour around England in the 1970s

Fat Man on a Bicycle, Tom Vernon, Fontana, London. An amusing, idiosyncratic account of travels on a bike by television's 'Fat Man'

Local Authority Cycle Routes List. Obtainable (enclose a SAE) from Cyclists' Touring Club (address above)

Penguin Book of the Bicycle, Watson and Gray, Penguin, Harmondsworth. A comprehensive, information-packed reference book.

Readers Digest Guide to Cycle Maintenance, Readers Digest, London. A very thorough guide

Round Ireland in Low Gear, Eric Newby, Collins, London. Wanda and Eric Newby's mountain-bike tour of Ireland, fuelled by Guinness and port. An entertaining and informative read

The Cycle Tourer's Handbook, Tim Hughes, Cyclists' Touring Club (address above). A useful reference book

4

Motoring in Retirement

Motoring in retirement is a different proposition from motoring when you're in full-time employment, although just how different depends on the role the car played in your job.

For instance, the car may have had nothing to do with your job at all—in which case the main difference will be that you will now have more time to use it for pleasure motoring than you did when your driving was restricted to weekends, evenings and holidays. On the other hand, you may have spent most of your working life in cars—in which case, in addition to a radical change in the sort of driving you do, you may also have to face up to the traumatic experience of having to hand in the company car. Between these two extremes there are any number of permutations but nothing is more certain than that retirement will bring some changes so it's as well to be prepared for them.

In some cases it might be worthwhile buying an interim vehicle a month or so before retirement day dawns, simply because the loss of the company car—often a cherished status symbol as well as a perk—appears at the time to be more of a deprivation than is usually the case, because although we know that in future we won't have to drive to work or cover huge business mileage it isn't easy to picture the reality. I relinquished the only company car I ever had many years ago so I know the feeling but—although I hadn't bought it for that reason—I did have an old jeep which saw me through until I was able to get another car.

Apart from that one job, which lasted only a few months, I've always had to find my own cars or do without and, almost without exception, they have been cars which no employer in his right mind would provide for his staff. From my elderly Lagonda to the hotted up Mini Cooper S—not to mention the Lancia, an Austin Healy 3000 and the rest—they were all fun motor-cars first and transport second. The point is that now you are no longer in full-time employment—

whether you have had a company car or not—your requirements will probably be very different and perhaps for the first time in your life you will be able to please yourself what sort of car you drive.

Choosing a Retirement Car

Up until recently, as an impulse buyer whose eyes light up at the sight of a gleaming bonnet or wire wheels, causing car dealers to rub their hands in gleeful anticipation, I wouldn't have been the one to advise on choosing which car to buy. However I'm now something of a reformed character and it is quite some time since I drove onto a dealer's forecourt in one car and off it in another.

I'm much more likely these days to take my time about choosing the right car, perhaps because I now appreciate that, apart from a house, a car is one of the largest single purchases most of us make; therefore, deciding what car to buy is very important. Money of course is a factor and although it may not be the problem we feared—for one thing instead of paying out on pensions and the like people now start paying us—some budgetting is usually essential.

However, let's forget money for the moment and ask ourselves about the sort of driving we've been doing in the past and the sort we shall be doing in the future. We could, of course, begin by asking ourselves if we are really going to need a car at all, especially if we live in town. It's possible that a month or so without a car could convince you that you don't need to buy one at all and that it's more economical just to hire one as needed, for long trips and holidays and so on.

Most of us, however, won't be ready for that sort of Draconian solution so we might go on to consider the sort of motoring we will almost certainly *not* be doing in the future.

Mileage
If we have used a car at all for business we shall now be doing considerably less mileage.

Speed
Time is no longer money in the sense that we could lose income or the boss's goodwill by being late for meetings or appointments. We can hand in our membership of the 'boy racers' club' and while we don't have to abandon the fast lane altogether it's no longer imperative that we live in it.

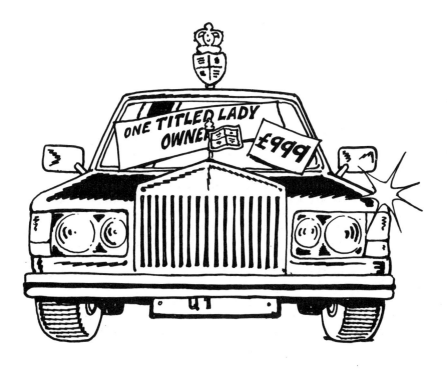

Sometimes there are genuine bargains to be had.

Prestige

Who cares? It's fun keeping up with the Jones's if we can afford it but on the other hand we can now allow ourselves to be thought a little eccentric because it's not going to affect our promotion or business prospects.

Load Capacity

Clients, samples, children—all no longer a problem. If you have longed for a two-seater all your life this could be the time to indulge yourself.

Reliability

Still important, but perhaps no longer vital; safety of course and good insurance are still as important as ever but no one is going to fire you if your car is off the road for a while.

Now that you have decided what sort of motoring you no longer *have* to do you could think about the motoring you would *like* to do.

You may, for instance, have to consider:

The Car for Shopping and Luggage Carrying

You may no longer have a family to consider so you won't need as much shopping capacity. However, you may now wish to do a week's or month's shopping in one trip, especially if you live out of town or travel to a hypermarket. At the same time, if you are going to travel in retirement, you will almost certainly want a fair amount of luggage space.

It's also worth remembering that sooner or later our ability to lift heavy weights out of car boots that look like linen chests is going to diminish, so try for a boot that opens flush with the bumper—or choose a hatchback.

Size

If you are buying new and have a partner, it's as well to remember that instead of long journeys with just the radio for company there will now usually be two of you so a very small economical car could feel cramped. It's a good idea to try out the different size models and discuss what you both feel about them.

If you are buying secondhand there's a lot to be said for a medium-size or even a large car. For one thing it's a lot more difficult to flog a larger car to death and besides, an expensive larger car is more likely to have been in private ownership and people do tend to treat their own machines with rather more care than they do other people's.

As a retired person you have the time to look for the real bargain—a largish car which is still as good as the day it left the factory but which has depreciated by many thousands of pounds.

Of course a big car will use more petrol than a small one—although even in the matter of fuel consumption retirement can bring advantages because hammering up and down the motorway at the sort of speeds favoured by working drivers can be very bad for your wallet. Most manufacturers will tell you what their cars will do at a constant 55 mph—which is very useful if you happen to live in America where the speed limit is an unbelievable 55 but not so useful for the ton-up gents in the fast lane in Britain. On the other hand it's quite a useful guide for people who have the time to take an off-motorway route or even to saunter along at 60 mph or so on the motorway. The other major disadvantage of a large and—when new—expensive car is that parts tend to be costly. However, unless the car is very old you can normally insure against any really nasty shocks in the first year of a secondhand car, which means that if you have bought wisely you should be okay. In any case you can buy an awful lot of extra petrol and new bits and bats for the thousands of pounds you will have saved. Besides, if you can't treat yourself to luxury motoring now you've retired—when will you be able to?

There's another advantage, too, in having a larger car, especially when you are getting older; if you should be unfortunate enough to have a shunt a bigger car gives you and your passengers more pro-tection—which, bearing in mind the fact that our bones are probably more brittle than when we were younger, is worth considering.

Of course, in the end, it all comes down to what you want in the way of motoring and what you can afford and if money is really tight the only people who can permit themselves to drive an old banger are the carefree youngsters and folks like us. Should you decide on the 'banger' option you could use the time you now have available to shop wisely and if you are not already a competent motor mechanic now is the time to enroll for a course in elementary maintenance.

Motoring Organisations

If you can afford it, whatever car you buy, you should consider joining a motoring organisation like the Royal Automobile Club (RAC) or the Automobile Association (AA). Both are invaluable for breakdown services, touring advice, travel information, maps, etc. Their hand-books, too, give details of a surprising range of services.

In my grandfather's day people seemed to be automatically mem-bers of both so that 'AA RAC' rolled off the tongue as one word. Nowadays it makes sense to choose one or the other. They offer pretty much the same service but stress different aspects. The RAC—they prefer just the initials these days—who have spent millions of pounds in recent years on new technology to improve their roadside service, pride themselves on their 'go not tow' policy which means that if it is possible to fix the car on the spot they'll fix it. Their patrol men keep their vehicles at home rather than at the depot so that off-duty men, they claim, can respond more quickly in case of a major emergency.

However, as a lifelong member of the AA I know quite a lot about them and, as Tony Court—who is one of their leading spokesmen—is a friend it seemed a good idea to pick his brains about driving in retirement, with special reference to motoring organisations. In this connection, although I've never been what you might call a 'joiner', I am becoming increasingly aware that, as you get a little older, joining clubs and other organisations can make a lot of sense, especially if the club's activity is something you haven't tackled before, like rambling or cycling. That way you get a lot of new, ready made, like minded acquaintances—some of whom could become friends—and all the facilities, plus a great deal of shared information—and if you are a rugged individualist you can always go it alone after your first sub runs out.

The AA is slightly different because, as Tony Court pointed out, joining the AA is a sort of insurance primarily against breaking down, whether at home or abroad, while for older people there is the added security of knowing that, should they by any chance fall ill, there is an air ambulance to whisk them home under medical supervision.

As a non-mechanical person I've always been a member of a motoring organisation, even when I could hardly afford a car and, to give them their due, they have never turned up their noses when called upon to get my real bangers moving. One patrolman, however, was sorely tried when he stopped, as he thought, to repair a Bentley I had hired for a newspaper chase and discovered that instead I wanted him to repair the elderly van I'd been chasing—to help me make friends with the quarry!

Basic membership is almost essential for most retired drivers and it is worthwhile considering the range of additional services on offer, but before doing this it's a good idea to find out exactly what you are entitled to as an ordinary member. Your personal membership entitles you to use of the 24-hour roadside service and if the patrolman can't get you going you get a free tow to the nearest AA recommended garage.

The average time taken by AA patrols to reach a breakdown—there are 3,400 patrolmen and they handle more than 3,000,000 calls a year—is 45 minutes. Motorway calls are relayed by the police from the roadside emergency phones, which can save you a small fortune if you have to join the unhappy band on the hard shoulder.

One minor plus point about being retired—but one which could prove very important—is that you now have the time to read through your AA handbook. Of course I've always found this publication invaluable—although I do wish they still sent it through the post instead of all the advertising mail—but, apart from using the gazetteer to find hotels and garages, I hadn't really read it through. This was silly of me because along with a lot of other valuable information and advice it tells you just what services you are entitled to. As Tony pointed out, retired people can get maximum benefit from the Travel Information Service. 'We can help by doing all the initial planning for any tours or trips at home or abroad, even when it comes to booking hotels.'

Maintenance

The AA reckon that more than one third of the breakdowns their patrol men deal with each year are caused by lack of elementary maintenance — things as simple as checking tyre pressures, putting in oil, water and of course petrol and making sure the battery is charged correctly.

If you have been spoiled up to now by having your company car serviced for you, now could be a good time to consider a course in basic maintenance. These are often held by the local Adult Education people but many technical colleges also run afternoon or evening courses and you'll often find that it's a popular choice for a course at a local community centre. Your council information office or one of the motoring organisations should be able to tell you of any local courses; if there isn't one in your area it might be an idea to suggest that the council starts one.

Preparation

When making a longish trip or travelling abroad it's a good idea to pay special attention to elementary maintenance but it also pays to service the car regularly or to have your local garage run the rule over it. The fact is that the car which has been pottering around happily on shopping excursions often isn't ready for a few thousand miles of autoroute or the backroads of rural Europe.

Take spares like plugs, bulbs and a warning triangle — you can get check lists of essentials from your motoring organisation — but a great deal depends on variables like the make of car so it's as well to make your own list. Molly's father, who invariably drove very old cars, rarely moved without enough spare parts to do a complete rebuild but then he was the sort of engineer who was happiest under a car bonnet.

Loading
Make sure your car is correctly loaded, especially if you use a roof rack; a badly loaded one can lead to real problems if stuff comes loose on a

motorway. This can be avoided by loading the roof rack moderately but don't transfer all the baggage to the car instead because over-loading the car itself can lead to trouble. Try instead to cut down on luggage a little and remember that if the spare wheel is beneath a mountain of gear it could ruin your trip should you have a puncture.

Tony Court recommends a practice run before embarking on a lengthy trip, especially if you intend motoring abroad. 'Pack everything you are going to take, exactly as you intend to pack it for the journey. That way you can make certain that the load hasn't affected the way your car drives.' This makes very good sense — and of course you now have the time for it.

Driving on the Continent

Driving on the Continent should cause no problems, especially as you will usually be able to take a scenic route which saves expensive toll fees as well as wear and tear on both you and the car and there's usually no need to book accommodation in advance except in the high season when it's essential to do so. If at all possible avoid the whole of the month of August which is when most of Europe seems to be racing for the Mediterranean and the Continent becomes one great traffic jam. It's also best to plan to avoid morning and evening rush hours in cities even if it means a long detour or spending a few hours exploring or having a good meal.

On the spot fines are high on the Continent and one suspects — without any proof whatsoever — that a car with GB plates and a Union Jack on the windscreen is more enticing game than a car with local number plates. As we now have time to observe all the rules we should be okay but it could be a good idea to make sure that some over-zealous 'flic' doesn't ruin your trip by taking some extra travellers cheques with you so that you can replace any cash they may relieve you of.

Driving in America

Driving in America is a pleasure because the whole place is built around the car, with long straight roads, plenty of convenient accommodation and — outside the big cities — reasonable parking.

Most visitors hire cars or rather 'rent' them — although if cash is a problem and you intend travelling long distances then car delivery is an option worth considering. Almost all hire cars are automatic so, if you have never driven one, either specify a 'stick shift' or get a few miles of practice on an automatic before you leave home. On my first trip to America I arrived in Florida and found to my horror that my rental car was an automatic which was something completely new to me. Added to that it was pouring with rain and pitch dark. Driving with one foot instead of two isn't something you really want to learn under those conditions and I was so busy trying not to change gear with the footbrake that I took a wrong turn out of the airport. America is a big country but I began to get worried when I realised that I hadn't seen a single light for a long time, never mind the bright lights of Palm Beach. Fortunately, just as I was beginning to panic, I came across a garage in the middle of nowhere where four huge and intimidating gentlemen—who I later discovered were of the type known as 'good ol' boys'—were so amused to find an Englishman driving purposefully into the swampland that they gave me a can of beer as well as first-class directions. When I reached my hotel the car started whining and I had to ask the hall porter what it was trying to tell me. It seems I'd left a door slightly open, which wasn't serious but it does show how important it is to familiarise yourself with your hired car and to find out not only how the gears work but where all the switches and levers are.

Ask the hire company staff to show you how everything works or you could find yourself indicating a turn with the windscreen wiper. American hire companies usually much prefer to show you how things work rather than let you drive away and have a shunt. However, it's important to have a good look at the hire car before you drive away. The vehicles are usually in good condition and if you do have problems all you need to do is to drive to the company's nearest office and they'll change the car without question rather than have you hanging around while they fix it, but if you take it back with a mark or a bump that you haven't pointed out to them then you are to blame. This close inspection is a bit difficult in torrential rain at midnight but if you do find a bump the following morning an immediate phone call to the company pointing out the circumstances is more likely to be sympathetically considered than the same explanation a couple of weeks later.

One important point is not to book in somewhere a long distance from the airport for your first night. Collecting the hire car may get you a bit worried about the time—especially if your plane is late—and you will find yourself rushing to get started instead of taking it easy and checking everything. Better to stay near the airport, you'll be in a much more relaxed mood the next day, which is the time to try out a new car in a new country.

If you are going to drive a long way it's worth asking if there are any special rules about crossing State lines—the Californians, for instance, get upset if you try to take in food and while I never got caught trying to smuggle in a beefburger I did have trouble with some special beer bought in one state for a barbecue we were having in the next State and discovered that we had inadvertently become bootleggers.

Some traffic rules vary from State to State but one which doesn't is the speed limit which is a yawn making 55 mph, rigidly enforced on everyone—except truck drivers—to the point where police helicopters will clock you racing along an empty road across the Nevada desert. In most places there isn't as much lane hopping as in Europe and overtaking on the inside is perfectly legal. Also legal in some States—Florida is one—is taking a right turn when the traffic lights are against you. Not all out of State Americans know this and if you learn the local rules you can enjoy joining in the symphony of car horns as some poor devil wonders why he is apparently being urged to break the law.

Don't follow the example of the local driver who perhaps has enough clout to get away with speeding—best do what most Americans do, which is to regard your car as a mobile sitting room from which to watch the scenery roll by.

Costs

Buying a car is a question of what you want and what you can afford but you can save yourself money by getting professional help and advice, especially when buying secondhand. And, as I've said, you can also save money in both the short term and long term by doing your own routine maintenance.

Where you can save money too is by taking the time to plan your route meticulously or by getting your motoring organisation to do it for you. Noting down the road numbers, the turns and junctions in large script on a flip over pad is a good idea. If you don't believe this will save you a fortune, Molly will be only too glad to tell you about the many thousands of unnecessary miles I have driven simply because I was certain I knew the way and was too pig-headed to turn back or stop and check the route. Mind you, this is not to say that you shouldn't get off the beaten track deliberately—in fact I'm all for it but it should at least be your choice.

Another way you can save cash when driving in retirement is to spend some time selecting one or more motoring companions because if cash is a consideration it makes no sense to use an expensive vehicle and costly fuel to transport one person or even two when the same car could easily take four or perhaps five. Splitting the cost is an important saving and you might also be able to share the driving.

However, it's not worth saving money if it means spending time with people you can't stand and if you make a list of 'people we could bear to spend time in the car with' it could turn out to be surprisingly short, so the best thing is to decide on possible companions and then go on a couple of day trips with them before embarking on a Continental tour. Of course if you are going to a fixed destination the others could perhaps hire a car once you have arrived but if you are the only driver you could find yourself in the position of chauffeur when all you want to do is to laze around.

One sure way of saving money is to drive well within your car's capabilities. That red line on your rev counter isn't there for decoration, so don't pile on the revolutions until the engine screams for mercy. Remember it's now your own car and fierce acceleration, tyre screeching take-offs and braking that stands the car on its bonnet are bound to cost you money in the end.

Motoring isn't what it used to be but perhaps one of the reasons why there didn't seem to be a lot of traffic on the road 30 or 40 years ago was that half the cars had broken down. Remember the days of punctures, inefficient batteries, oil guzzling engines and cars that either wouldn't stop at all or performed gracious pirouettes whenever you touched the brakes in the wet? Remember too those days when you were driving too far and too fast in all sorts of weather conditions for 'business reasons'? Forget the good old days! In a modern car with much better reliability and performance than most old-time luxury cars, your driving in retirement should be some of the most comfortable and enjoyable motoring you have ever had.

Useful Tips

1. Keep the numbers of your car keys in your purse or wallet so they can easily—and cheaply—be replaced if lost
2. Don't overload the car with non-essential luggage
3. Plan your route carefully and keep maps and any addresses and telephone numbers of *en route* accommodation together in a plastic folder
4. Take regular rests to stretch your legs
5. Pack an emergency flask and food even for a short journey—food and drink are very comforting if there's a delay
6. Keep a good torch and a small first-aid kit in the glove compartment
7. Keep a spare pair of shoes and socks/stockings handy in case you step out into a puddle
8. Keep a cheap thin plastic mac with hood handy—even for the dash from car park to hotel

Useful Addresses

Automobile Association, Fanum House, Basingstoke, Hampshire. Telephone (0256) 20123

Disabled Drivers' Association, Ashwellthorpe, Norwich NR16 1EX. Telephone (050) 841 324. Branches throughout Britain—expert advice on mobility problems, vehicle adaptations, etc. Details of reduced rates for foreign travel, advice on holiday facilities. The Association owns its own hotel, at Ashwellthorpe, a fully-adapted country mansion

Royal Automobile Club, Lansdowne Road, Croydon CR9 2JA. Telephone (01) 686 2525

Further Reading

AA Guides, Automobile Association (address above). These are a series of guides, on Hotels, Restaurants, Guest Houses, Farmhouses, Inns, etc. Very informative on prices and facilities in all regions of Britain

Exchange and Mart. Weekly newspaper. The motoring supplement in particular is very useful for price comparisons of spare parts, secondhand cars, etc.

Shell Guide to Viewpoints of England, Garry Hogg, Osprey Philip. An unusual guide for the motorist who also likes walking; 15 circular maps with a high 'viewpoint' at the centre of each. An informative text accompanies the maps

Motorists' First Aid, British Red Cross, London. A useful A to Z of emergency care. Small enough to fit into the glove compartment

Travellers' France, Arthur Eperon, Croom Helm, London. An informative and detailed guide to touring in France, including the offbeat places. By the same author and publisher *Encore Travellers' France* is useful too

What Car?. A monthly magazine with the latest in motoring news, car assessments, etc. Obtainable from newsagents

Your Car. A monthly magazine for the car enthusiast—maintenance, expert advice, motoring news, etc. Obtainable from newsagents

5

The Not So
Raggle-Taggle Gypsies

If you have spent your working life in a job which entailed travelling, one of the major shocks of retirement is the fact that other people no longer pay your hotel bills.

Of course you've always realised that hotels are expensive but there's a lot of difference between grumbling as you sign the bill for an overnight stay and actually having to fork out for bed and breakfast from your own pocket. The realisation that last night's gourmet dinner is no longer going to be covered by expenses can change one's attitude towards quite a few things—and caravans in particular.

I have to admit that in my expense account heyday I regarded caravans as a nuisance and a driving hazard which appeared as if by magic whenever I was in a hurry. I couldn't understand why Molly's father, otherwise a rational sort of chap with a genuine liking for cars, should acquire one of the things almost as soon as he retired from his full-time job. It didn't even occur to me to wonder how, on a limited income, he was able to spend several months a year either in Spain or the South of France, not to mention taking half a dozen or so extended trips to various parts of the British Isles.

Of course the time for my conversion should have come when Harry died and we were offered the caravan as a gift but, being a total idiot, I declined with thanks; I didn't fancy driving along with one of those things attached to my car, slowing me down to a crawl and playing Hell with my image.

It was only at a later date that I began to realise that Harry had found an ideal way of travelling in retirement. It was then that I became aware that ever since I met her, Molly had been extolling the virtues of caravanning—the economy, the freedom and so on—only to be told, each time she brought up the subject, that our current car was much too good for towing and that I was too big and too tall to live in a mobile doll's house.

Now I have been forced to rethink my attitude towards caravans—

45

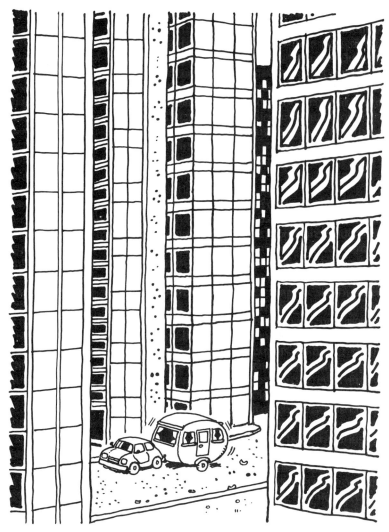

Nowadays it can be easier to find an official camp site.

for the cash saving alone—and I've had to admit that she and her parents were right all along but, to give her her due, she has never once said 'I told you so!'

Of course things have changed a lot since Harry's caravanning days and it is no longer quite so easy to set off into the blue and be sure of finding a friendly farmer wherever you care to stop. Today, even free spirits like my friend Patrick Leal tend to use caravan sites, both for safety and convenience and since Pat is an all year round caravanner he should know what he's doing. In many ways, apart from the fact that he has no other home, Pat is a typical caravanner in retirement and as he is 60-years-old and not in the best of health his total enjoyment of caravanning indicates that it is something almost anyone can tackle. Pat is perhaps atypical in one way in that, as a former aircraft engineer, he has little trouble in keeping his 2 litre 1971 Mercedes in good fettle and has been able to refit his own van, which was a considerable saving. He paid £220 in 1984 for the Cheltenham Puku four-berth van, since when he has virtually rebuilt the interior which now has a hint of ship's cabin about it.

'It has good cooking facilities and the standard caravan toilet fittings — which I rarely use because if you stay at Caravan Club sites all the time, as I do, you have your toilet block with showers and everything. I pay the annual fee for my Caravan Club membership which means, among other things, that every time I stay at a site it's cheaper than it would be otherwise. All in all it costs me between £20 and £22 a week — that's for me, my van, toilet facilities, heating, hot water and so on — everything except food and petrol.'

For those who don't want to spend all year in the their van, caravanning is yet another means of travel which offers financial advantages to retired people as the rates charged by camp sites both here and abroad vary according to the season. Not having to travel at peak times means that the roads are less crowded and sites not only cheaper but more readily available.

'I don't have any other home.' says Pat cheerfully. 'There's no point — after all you can't sit in two chairs at once and if I want to go anywhere I take my home with me. I've got the van just the way I like it. If there's a power cut in winter I can switch to gas heating, using Propane gas, but normally my two bar electric fire keeps me very cosy indeed and my heating bills are nothing like they would be in a house. I do some cooking but I usually eat one meal out. There are a lot of working men's cafes about where you can get a damned good meal cheaply — with a choice of roast beef, lamb, pork and so on. I use caravan sites for convenience; they handle the refuse disposal, there are proper toilets and washing facilities. They save a tremendous amount of messing about, access is easy and you know that even in winter you will have no trouble getting on and off a site.'

The sites Patrick uses are operated by the Caravan Touring Club (CTC) which has been going for some 80 years and now has 181 sites and a membership of 262,000 families — which makes it the largest organisation of its kind in the world. Of the larger sites, 17 are in National Parks, 9 on land leased from the National Trust and 6 on Forestry Commission Land. There are 7 on large estates like

Sandringham and Longleat and in addition to the large sites there are more than 4,500 'Certified Locations'—small five-van sites exclusive to club members and situated mainly on farms.

These sites are about the closest you can get these days to the total freedom enjoyed by Molly's parents but it's probably as well to start with a larger site with all amenities if you are a beginner. In fact, it's almost certainly better to begin caravanning in your own driveway—but of course you first have to choose an outfit and, fortunately, being retired gives you the time to select a van, learn how to handle it at leisure and discover how to live in it.

Choosing a Rig

Matching a caravan with a suitable tow car is one of the most difficult problems caravanners face. However, caravanners who are retired people are unlikely to need a large multi-berth caravan—unless they are a soft touch as holiday baby-sitters—which does make things easier. The problem is that, as every solo motorist knows, caravanners can upset other road users and endanger themselves and others in two ways; by being or appearing to be unsafe and by holding up traffic. Being unsafe results from having a caravan too heavy for the tow car to handle safely; holding up traffic stems from having a tow car which doesn't have the power to pull almost twice its own weight.

Patrick's elderly Mercedes, he says, will pull his four-berth van up hill and down dale at 70 mph—or would do if the legal limit were not 60 mph. Living in his van all year he found a four-berth almost a must. He doesn't care for awnings but they have come a long way since the early rough and ready efforts and are now easily erected separate rooms with built in flooring, which makes it quite possible to use a smaller van—even if, like us, you are on the large size.

In fact a small van pulled by a heavy powerful car is ideal and I like the Rover 3.5 litre which is heavy, powerful, comfortable and has a good load carrying capacity. The point is that the more you can load into the car without unbalancing it and the less in the caravan the more secure you will be on the road. Something like the Rover is also relatively cheap to buy secondhand and you can buy an awful lot of petrol for the couple of thousand quid you could save on the purchase price.

However, if you feel you must have a small economical car for everyday use then it's compromise time. Aim for a towed weight of 85 per cent of the car's weight and never exceed 100 per cent—always remembering that the towed weight is the actual laden weight (ALW), that is, the empty weight of your caravan plus whatever you put in it. As a rule of thumb establish your caravan's ALW and multiply it by 1.2 as a guide to the kerb weight (KW) of car to aim for.

A similar rule of thumb for working out the power-to-weight ratio, which is almost as important as the weight relationship of car to van, is to aim for 40 bhp to every ton of 'train weight', which means everything your car has to pull i.e. your loaded car plus your loaded caravan—not forgetting yourselves.

Be careful if you own a diesel car, or are thinking buying one; they produce less power for the size of the engine—which means that the manufacturer's towing limit may be less than for petrol versions.

An automatic is ideal for towing because you can crawl where necessary without clutch slip and there is less wear and tear on the transmission. Automatics are also easier to operate than manual cars, especially when restarting on hills and reversing to hitch up, which makes it worthwhile putting up with their higher fuel consumption.

Whatever car you choose make sure the type of towing bracket you buy has been tested to British (AU 114) or International (ISO 3853) standards. It isn't worth trying to save a couple of pounds by buying an untested bracket so insist that the one you fit has a name and plate stating that the model has been tested to the required standard. Talking of towing brackets, one thing that even some experienced caravanners never seem to remember is that it's easier to take the car to the van than the van to the car. Said Patrick, 'They don't seem to realise that a car has an engine and the van hasn't.'

Making Friends with your Caravan

One slight drawback about being retired is that without even being aware of it we may well have become set in our ways—in which case the change to living in a caravan, even for fairly short periods, can be quite traumatic. As usual Pat Leal has the answer, which is quite simply to live in the caravan in your own driveway and if you can borrow or hire a model similar to the one you intend buying, so much the better. Says Patrick, 'I'd certainly advise people who take up caravanning for the first time when they retire to get in as much practice as possible in their own garden before setting off on a trip. As soon as they get a van, the first thing they should do is to park it by the side of the house, decide what they want to put in it from the weight point of view and then move in. They should live in the van as they would on a field or camp site, practising driving round the block, backing in, uncoupling, setting up, putting up the awning, getting the water, plugging in the electrics, turning on the gas and, with the exception of the toilet, not using the house facilities at all. By doing that for a couple of days you can iron out any little snags—and if you are retired you have the time to do it.'

'Don't forget that a holiday on a static caravan site is not the same as using a touring van of your own because holiday vans are all set up when you arrive. You need to learn how to get into a parking space, how to unhook—get right into a routine. If you can back a car you can back a caravan; just remember that the wheel goes in the opposite direction and never pull a caravan around when you've got the car to do it for you.'

Loading

There is a temptation—especially on the distaff side—to regard the caravan as a heaven-sent extra large suitcase but this should be resisted at all costs as the aim is to have as little as possible in the van.

Fortunately, being retired does give you the time to make lists, to pare down your luggage requirements and to practise packing and unpacking. For instance, water is very heavy—a gallon of water weighs ten pounds—so a couple of plastic squash bottles in the car should suffice for the essential cup of tea.

Make sure that gas bottles are upright and securely held and that breakables are stored where they won't come loose. Lash everything down as if for a storm at sea and you won't go far wrong. Incidentally we've discovered some excellent plastic crockery and I've even learned to live with plastic wine 'glasses'.

Molly's parents used to pull their Sprite van with a tremendous tank-like Austin Westminster and I remember being surprised at the way they packed every inch of space behind the front seats and in the huge boot, as well as putting a lot of stuff in front of my mother-in-law's feet and a huge amount of gear on the roof rack. I didn't realise at the time that they were following the first rule of loading a caravan which is—not to.

Essentials

A lot depends on whether you are going away for the weekend, a short tour in Britain or an extended trip abroad. The Caravan Club have a check list but it is probably better, as you have the time, to make your own. Caravan Club experts do suggest that once you have established your basic caravan requirements you should leave them in the van—otherwise you may arrive on site short of something essential like a corkscrew.

Leave the chip pan at home! It's a fire hazard for everyone but especially for those of us whose reactions have slowed down a touch. If you must have chips then buy them from a shop, have them with a restaurant meal or get a packet of 'oven ready' ones which you can heat up.

Starting Off

Make a check list to be gone through before setting off—if you have a partner you can play airline pilots and tick off each item before moving off! Then comes the great moment and, as one Caravan Club pamphlet puts it, 'First time caravanning is dotted with small but pleasing delights', the first being that the adjustment to towing a caravan is much easier than one might imagine.

In several important ways retired people have the advantage over other caravan users in that they can for example, pick the day they want to travel and the time of day. They have no need of a fast route or even to hurry. This doesn't mean that we have to dawdle but it does mean that we can duck into a handy lay-by if we find ourselves leading a procession and that we can be patient about overtaking, which is essential with a caravan when the TED or 'Time Exposed to Danger' is longer than in a solo car.

Courses

If you can afford the cash you can almost certainly afford the time to take one of the practical courses run by the Caravan Club. These include instruction on hitching up, towing safely and efficiently, understanding loading and how it affects towing, practice in manoeuvring an outfit forwards and backwards, simple mechanical and electrical principles, straightforward safety checks and the law as it affects caravanners. The course takes ten hours over one and a half days and normally has one instructor to every six students.

They even provide a caravan so all you have to do is to arrive in a car fitted with a towing bracket, functional electrics and two outside mirrors. You also have to know the kerbweight of your car, which you can find in the manual, and to possess a current driving licence. To my mind this is money well spent and you can even take a course before you invest in a caravan although you have to book well in advance as the courses are very popular.

A useful sequence for those beginning caravanning might be: (a) to stay in a holiday van; (b) take a caravanning course; (c) purchase a van; (d) practise setting up, driving round the block and living in the van at home; (e) take short trips, building up to a couple of weeks' stay, until several hundred miles of ordinary roads have been covered;

51

(f) begin motorway travelling. You should then be able to tackle anything, including foreign travel.

Breakdown Insurance

It makes sense to insure your car and caravan as comprehensively as you can, not forgetting that there are clothes, equipment and other contents to be covered. Consult your current motor insurance company or check with the Caravan Club who, in addition to insuring your van, will advise on security and will also register your van's chassis number on their computer.

The Caravan Club also run a Mayday Caravan Rescue Service for roadside repair and recovery which offers all-year-round protection even without your caravan—which means you are covered for ordinary motoring as well. I was interested to learn that Pat Leal, who as a former matelot and aircraft engineer could probably repair Concorde with a nail file and a couple of elastic bands, is a Mayday subscriber.

There are three packages: the comprehensive package gives you complete breakdown service even for flat tyres and is a boon for the older non-mechanical types like me. They'll even bring you petrol if you run out. If you have an accident or a major breakdown they will get you, your car, your caravan and up to five passengers home and take your car to the nearest garage—or they'll take you on to your nearest destination. There's also a £6 'extra protection' package which takes care of everything, including getting you and all your rig home if you are too ill to drive and provides legal aid if needed and also helps with hotel accommodation. Home calls are also offered as an optional extra.

Roadside Assistance, costing £19 with optional home call, offers speedy assistance to deal with minor faults or will transport the complete rig and passengers to the nearest approved garage if the fault can't be put right at the roadside.

Recovery—the third option—is for people who are able to tackle minor roadside repairs themselves and for £16.75 will make sure that if you have a major breakdown you, your rig and passengers will be taken back home or on to your destination.

There was a time when I was a 'third party, fire and theft' man, partly because I couldn't afford any other sort of insurance, but those were the days when road travel was an adventure, when lorry drivers were knights of the road and even garage men occasionally took pity on the hopeless and hapless. Now, sad to say, juggernaut drivers haven't time to see you, never mind stop and help, while most filling station staff know only enough about mechanics to operate a till. That being the case, if you know as much about mechanical things as I do then £39 for a comprehensive roadside repair, nationwide recovery and home call service, plus illness and legal aid protection, makes sense.

Caravanning in Europe

Patrick, who never does things by halves, recently made a leisurely eight month tour of Spain, France, Germany and the Benelux countries. 'It was great—I just got a green card and bought myself a few bail bonds for the countries where I knew I might need them.'

'In Spain, for instance, if you have any sort of trouble or are involved in an accident, the police are inclined to throw everyone in jail while they sort it out. If you have a bail bond you are let out on bail but if not you could be in jail for three months or so while they deal with things. For the sake of a pound or two on top of the Green Card it's not worth the risk.'

Pat found that costs varied but, on the whole, European touring worked out cheaper than touring in England because the food was cheaper. 'Where in England can you get a decent steak with a couple of eggs and all the trimmings, washed down with a beer, ice-cream to follow and a brandy with your coffee, all for a couple of quid like you can in Germany? The Continent used to be dear by comparison with England but that isn't the case anymore and, in Spain especially, food and drink are still very reasonable indeed.' Pat admits that having been a sailor and a world traveller before retiring helps a lot but insists that anyone can learn to tour with a caravan, both at home and abroad.

Most European roads are good and, once again, travelling in retirement means that you can save money and stress by not travelling in the high season, in addition to which the sites themselves tend to be much less crowded. As we mentioned in the last chapter, the month of August is definitely the time to avoid the Continent as the roads are jammed with cars rushing to and from the Mediterranean. We spent nearly six months on a site in the South of France and were quite upset when the summer people came down to invade our 'privacy' in July and August—especially as we then had to pay more anyway.

Although you'll have the time to take the longer routes there will be occasions when you want to use the direct road and if you've done a few hundred miles on British motorways you should be ready for the autobahns, the autoroutes and the autostradas—not to mention the highways and by-ways of Europe, but do read up on road signs before you set off.

For your first venture it might be worthwhile considering one of the inclusive foreign trips which include car ferry costs, insurance, site fees for specified locations, some meals and lots of directories and maps, plus a certain amount of discreet shepherding. After that you should feel confident to make your own way and there are a lot of good site guides to help you choose your route. The advantage of using Caravan Club sites is that they have been tried and tested and have usually been the subject of members' reports over the years, but this shouldn't stop you looking out for places where the beauty of the location may make up for the lack of facilities. With your temporary 'home' behind your car you can try out such places for a night or two and may even find that they are more to your taste.

Caravanettes

I've always fancied a caravanette but serious caravanners like Pat Leal shake their heads whenever you mention them because, they say, most of them are underpowered and are difficult to park anywhere in towns, whereas a tow car needs only to be unhitched to provide normal transport.

The advantage is that you don't have to bother unhitching a caravanette. If you intend using your mobile holiday home simply to drive to a holiday site and stay there—perhaps using bicycles for transport—then a caravanette could be for you, but if you want to have motorised transport when you arrive, and don't want the expense of hiring, then a towed caravan is the answer. There is also a fairly common complaint from caravanette owners that if they go off for the day, even if they have booked and paid for a site, their place is often occupied when they return. Even if this is eventually sorted out it can be very frustrating to find another family *in situ*, especially when it's late and you are tired and dying for a meal.

To be fair, though, these car homes have become much more sophisticated than they once were and, in general, the engines have been uprated so if you can afford a new one you'll find that some of them are very good indeed. As I mentioned, you might consider solving the mobility problem by taking bicycles with you, a principle which has been taken to its logical conclusion by some American motor-home owners who even pull their cars behind them on special trailers. Mind you, they do travel vast distances and in a country which is geared to huge vehicles, as well as having thousands of trailer parks.

So, before you decide on anything large in the way of caravanettes it's as well to imagine yourself trying to get it through the narrow lanes of a small English town on market day before you venture further afield.

Cost

Cost is a 'How long is a piece of string' question. You can pay anything for an outfit, from a few hundred pounds to the £50,000 some Americans and Arabs are prepared to spend. By and large, with new cars and vans, you get what you pay for although it's worthwhile using the time you now have at your disposal to shop around for exactly what you want and for the best bargain.

Experienced caravanners advise first hiring an outfit most like the one you intend buying and, if you are buying new, this could save a lot of grief. A few days will sort out whether you need a size smaller or larger and whether the layout of a particular van suits you and if you are comfortable towing it.

With secondhand vans—or outfits if you are starting from scratch —the choice and price range is immense but, assuming you are looking for economy and are prepared to take your time, there are some real bargains to be picked up. Many caravans—and some, but very much fewer, cars—are hardly used over the years, which means that if they have been reasonably maintained they should be very nearly as new. There really are 'little old ladies' around who occasionally sell cars and caravans and fortunately those of us with time at our disposal can spend a day or two sorting out the genuine bargains from the rubbish.

Meanwhile, to give an idea of the sort of things available at the bargain basement end of the market, keep an eye on the classified section of your local newspaper. There you will find advertisements like, for example: '1974 14 ft caravan with a double bed and a single, complete with full awning, for sale. £750'; '10 ft four-berth caravan for sale, £475. Includes toilet and gas bottle. Very good condition, fitted with an expensive stabiliser.' People who have already spent money, as this last ad indicates, on improving what you intend buying are always good news. But beware other ads; for example, a caravan from a country district could mean that it has been well used even though it might appear a bargain. Search out the advertisements for a trailer tent. This gives you another option when it comes to cheap and cheerful accommodation and has the great advantage of being easy to tow. People will often sell utensils when they decide to sell the tent, so look for adverts such as 'trailer tent with kitchen sink, cooker and many extras'.

One difficulty does present itself with tents. Unlike caravan awnings, which are a luxury, tents have to be erected as soon as you reach your destination, whatever the weather. Of course, they do sleep quite a few so if you are in a position to offer a cheap holiday to two or three younger members of the family who happen to be Scouts or the like, and who are well able to get on with putting up the tent while you recce the local amenities, it could be a good way of travelling in retirement. However, if there are just two of you, or if you are travelling solo and at times of year and in countries where the weather cannot be relied on, then a caravan is warmer, cosier and more convenient.

Molly's parents, incidentally, turned their very ordinary van into a luxurious model by making new curtains and loose covers and fitting a good quality carpet. As covers are often standard issue these additions can make a surprising difference to the appearance and comfort of the caravan.

Whatever you choose, you'll need a car—if you haven't already got one— and, as we've mentioned, preferably a fairly powerful one. Again, look to the classifieds! They may well advertise just the sort of tow car bargain that retired people like you have the time to check out. Say, 'Humber Sceptre 1975 in excellent condition inside and out, taxed, long MOT, with sunshine roof and (wait for it) only 35,000 miles on the clock. On offer at £425.' Okay, I'm an optimist with a touching faith in human nature but there *really are* people who buy cars new and then use them just for shopping and a couple of long trips a year. So, it is just possible in this case. The Humber would tow a small caravan at legal motorway speeds for ever and, at that mileage—if genuine—would be barely run in.

By shopping around for similar bargains—and getting them checked out if you are not mechanically minded—you could be on the road with a car and caravan for about £900—say £1,000 if the car needed fitting with a towbar.

Additional Costs

Membership of the Caravan Club, as Patrick Leal showed us earlier, is an essential, at least for beginners. It costs very little per year plus a joining fee and a nominal extra payment for each family member.

Insurance, of course, depends on the size and value of your outfit while Get-You-Home services and so on are optional but well worth thinking about for peace of mind.

Site fees depend very much on the nature of the site and the time of year but, on a well-equipped site, will average out very reasonably and will include electricity though there will be extra charges for any additional occupants.

If you can afford the original investment—double it if you need to buy a car as well—then living in a caravan especially for a couple, could work out a lot cheaper than the most reasonable orthodox accommodation. For retired people this sort of saving is extremely important as it could well mean the difference between going on holiday for a meagre fortnight or so and travelling for perhaps a couple of months or more a year.

Come to think of it, the temptation to flog the house and do a

Patrick Leal by taking to the open road with a few thousand quid in my pants back pocket is a very real one, but one which Molly, perhaps fortunately, has so far found herself able to resist on my behalf!

Useful Addresses

American Independence Travel, 6 Clarence Terrace, Warwick Street, Leamington Spa, Warwickshire. Camper and motor-home rentals throughout America

International Camper Exchange, PO Box 5794, Bellevue, WA 98006, America

International Register, Changing Wheels, CW House, 88 Fallowcourt Avenue, London N12 0BG

Motor Camper Rentals International, PO Box 11, Halesowen, West Midlands

The Caravan Club, East Grinstead House, East Grinstead RH19 1UA. Telephone (0342) 26944

Further Reading

Caravan. A monthly magazine, obtainable from newsagents

Caravanning. A monthly magazine obtainable from newsagents

Exchange and Mart. A weekly newspaper with a section devoted to caravan sales

6

Plain Sailing in Retirement

Or How Not to Mess About in Boats

'Messing about in boats' is a phrase with a seductive ring to it for those of us who are no longer in full-time employment, evoking as it does carefree sunny days on the water, while at the same time hinting at a maritime heritage in a way which somehow combines idleness with virtue.

The fact is though that, when it comes to boats, messing about is the sort of thing that could seriously abridge your retirement and the only sailors who can afford to adopt a relaxed attitude towards water are those who know exactly what they are doing. This doesn't mean that sailing can't be enjoyable — most forms of water travel are fun and many are ideal for older people — but it does mean that water has to be treated with respect.

I learned this the hard way recently when I did some canoeing for my book *Beginners Luck* without having time to take a proper course in how to handle the thing. I saw myself in imagination, muscles rippling under fringed buckskins as I paddled my fur laden canoe up some remote Canadian river; in reality however I was rather too plump for canoeing at the time, with the result that when I capsized — which was almost inevitable — I became the keel of a keel-less boat and a fixed keel at that as, in my panic, I had forgotten about the quick release toggle and was stuck upside down in the water like a cork in a bottle. Fortunately, after swallowing rather a lot of the Avon in an attempt to dog paddle to the surface while still attached to the canoe, I remembered what I had been told and got free. As it happened a lot of help was very near at hand so only my pride was in danger. Even so, my instructors stressed that had I not been in a hurry to write the story there was no way they would have allowed me on the river at that stage — let alone down the weir that I went over after my fifth capsize — before giving me a complete course of instruction in the

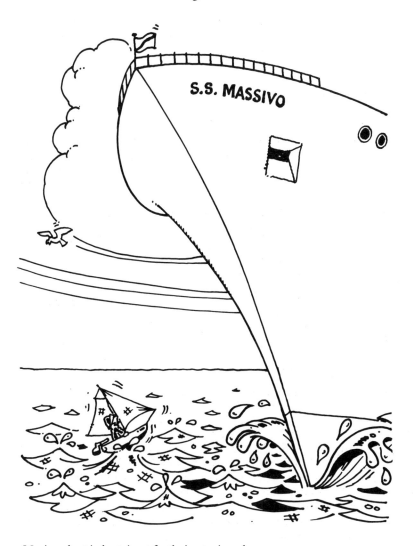

Messing about in boats is not for the inexperienced.

safety of a swimming bath.

I'd learned my lesson and it was one that was confirmed when I tried other forms of sailing and boating, namely that if you want to travel on water, other than as a passenger, it's essential to get instruction from a suitably experienced and preferably qualified person.

For most of us, water is an unfamiliar and sometimes unforgiving element so, at the risk of seeming po-faced and unadventurous, I'd say that everyone who wants to take up any kind of sailing, especially if they are close to or over retiring age, should join an appropriate club and take lessons. In fact I'd go further and suggest that if you want to take up any form of water sport and can't swim it would be a good idea to learn. There was a time when most sailors refused to learn to swim, preferring a quick demise to a slow one, but since few of us will be doing much trans-Atlantic rowing their reasoning doesn't apply and being able to do even a few strokes might be handy.

Apart from the obvious advantages of being able to get back in the boat, should we fall in, being able to swim is a marvellous confidence builder and a useful way of getting to know something about how water behaves when we move about, either in it or on it. That being said, if you do join a sailing club you'll find the members so safety conscious you'll begin to suspect that they're desperate not to lose your subscription because they just won't let you come to any harm. Not only that but most experienced sailing folk combine a missionary zeal in recruiting newcomers to their hobby with a great deal of patience when it comes to passing on their skills.

Clubs are Trumps

The good news is that there are as many types of clubs as there are ways of travelling on water and nearly all of them are prepared to welcome inexperienced older people with open arms. The even better news is that hundreds of these clubs are affiliated to the Royal Yachting Association (RYA). Among the many other benefits the Association offers, it will help you to find a club which exactly suits your needs. Joining the RYA is money well spent, especially if you are thinking of sailing in retirement. This is because the RYA covers all forms of sailing from wind-surfing to speedboats, luxury yachts and for that matter fully rigged sailing ships and can therefore help you to choose the sort of sailing you want to do.

Of course we are talking about travel in retirement but dinghy sailing will certainly be a help in learning to manage a larger yacht, while learning to handle any sort of powered craft will make you more proficient when it comes to, say, a cabin cruiser.

What Sort of Sailing?

Most of us will not be going in for long-distance board sailing, or be thinking of taking a dinghy across the Atlantic—and those of us who do will probably know exactly what they are doing anyway. We can also forget about those whose idea of sailing in retirement is to buy a luxury yacht—except to warn them to be careful how they choose their crew.

Between the Marine Commando type of sailing and the pampered life of a luxury yacht owner there is a vast range of water travel which older non-millionaires can enjoy and for the dedicated sailor a life afloat can be surprisingly economical.

Our friend John Gardner, for example, is 66-years-old and a retired theatre manager, stage manager and props manager whose working life left him richer in memories than in money. He's also lame, a fact which I didn't discover until the first time we left his boat to walk down to the pub when I realised that on dry land he finds it easier to use a crutch. John and his wife Zena, who was usually in charge of wardrobe where John was working, bought the *Lyreen*, a 32 ft motor-sailor for £8,000 in 1982 and although it would be worth quite a bit more now—mainly because of the work they've done—the price would be much closer to that of a mobile home or a largish motor-home than that of a house or flat.

As it is, their floating home has a forward cabin with three bunks, one of which they use for storage, a main saloon which also has three bunks, a galley, a toilet and a washroom. Mooring fees vary but they pay around £75 a month for the average marina mooring which includes water, a private car park with toilet and shower block and, while they do pay extra for electricity which is charged at commercial rates, they find they don't use a lot.

Of course John and Zena don't just travel from marina to marina but while they love going to places like St Ives in Cornwall, where the tide goes out and they can walk ashore, they find that mooring out in most harbours where they have to row in every time they want to go ashore is a bit tiring so they favour marinas if they are going to be in a place for any length of time. John is convinced that almost anyone retiring at 60 or 65 could take up sailing. 'It all depends what they want to do. I now insist on a motor sailor which has plenty of engine so I haven't got a lot of clambering about on decks to do. If anything happens to the engines I've at least got a sail I can bring us in with, but unless the weather is absolutely perfect for sails, for us, are just an emergency thing. Unless you are hopping across the Channel you've no need to sail out of sight of land and we tend to work our way round the coast, calling into our favourite ports on the way. We always sail during the day. Sailing at night is too much like hard work for older people; you can't see anything, which means you have to do all the ship work with someone at the helm and you can't sleep. We have a VHF radio abroad—I wouldn't sail without one—but we haven't got radar because we can't afford it. I'd like it though and I think that now merchant ships rely on satellite navigation—which means that light-houses are disappearing—it's going to be essential.'

The Gardners's boat does around seven knots and gets through one third of a gallon an hour, which means they can get around 20 miles to the gallon—not at all bad for an engine that's half a century old.

Like most retired people who have become sailors John and Zena appreciate the fact that their preferred means of travel also takes them close to inexhaustible supplies of free food. 'We drop a net over the side sometimes and catch a couple of pounds of prawns. We got a shock when we priced them recently and discovered that we'd eaten about £4 for supper one night.' Fishing can in fact save quite a bit of money and the fact that many experts consider fish to be the ideal defence against heart disease could be an added bonus, while—as I discovered many years ago—any surplus fish you catch can readily be converted into pocket money or beer, depending on whether your friends are professional fishermen or landlords of pubs.

The Gardners, whose boat is extremely snug and warm, usually lie up for the winter but when they are on the South Coast they go out fishing, even in winter, to supplement their diet—and their income.

The Cost of Freedom

The Gardners paid £8,000 for their boat, which is not too much for a home but is a lot for a hobby. They find it as cheap to live in as a house; once they have paid their marina fees they have no rates or water rates to find and of course there are still places where the mooring is free, as well as a number of bays where you can drop anchor.

Taking a boat the size of the *Lyreen* out of the water for maintenance and putting it back is expensive so John prefers to get somewhere where he can wait till the tide goes out, enabling him to climb underneath and do what needs to be done himself. Maintenance costs and repairs depend enormously on what sort of boat you have but, bearing in mind the sort of money you have to pay painters and mechanics, the more you can do yourself the better it is. Now that you're no longer just a weekend sailor trying to relax after the pressures of work you can enjoy taking your time getting the boat ready for your travels.

Incidentally, the Gardners always radio the Coast Guard or tell the Harbour Master when they are leaving port, where they intend to go and, if possible, their Estimated Time of Arrival (ETA) and as soon as they get into port they report, 'Here we are—we've arrived safely'.

'We used to feel they wouldn't want to be bothered with silly old pensioners like us always calling in,' said John 'but we've discovered that in fact they are only too pleased that we do so.'

Sailing the Waterways

Last time I spoke to them the Gardners were planning to take their boat through the French canal system and down to Portugal where they intend making their base for a while. They'll find that the French have organised private inland waterway travel for a lot longer than the British have, which means, paradoxically, that there seem to be fewer restrictions on things like mooring, and, except for fuel costs, canal travel is cheaper in France.

In Britain it was beginning to look as though the waterways would become un-navigable through neglect but the leisure boom of the last few years has changed all that. Today the British Waterways Board (BWB) own, or are the navigating authority for, a network of nearly 2,000 miles of waterways, mainly man-made canals and rivers suitable for navigation.

If you become hooked on travelling the waterways you'll probably want to own your own boat and perhaps live on it for part of the year or even on a more or less permanent basis but before spending the sort of money that entails it's just as well to find out if it's really the sort of thing you'll enjoy.

Fortunately, the BWB—which is divided up into seven geographical areas for England and Wales plus five areas for Scotland—has exactly the thing for a trial run, an excellent scheme for all-in holidays afloat which includes Canal Breakaways of up to five days. This scheme is an ideal introduction, especially for retired people who can benefit from low season and weekday rates as opposed to the more expensive times. At their base in Nantwich the BWB also run Open Days which provide a chance to inspect their narrow boats.

Up until recently the main difficulty for retired people was that most narrow boats for hire were from four- to eight-berth which meant that a couple who wanted to travel on their own faced the same expense as a family group. Of course this is still an option if a group of you want to holiday together but now, for the first time, there's a Water Sable Class two- to three-berth boat available. Hire costs vary according to season, but its ease of handling makes it popular with beginners.

Barges for Beginners

Almost anyone can handle a narrow boat, whatever their age, but while a visit to the Open Day or a 'phone call to Nantwich may have relieved any doubts on this score you may still find the idea of making your own way in an unfamiliar craft a bit daunting. Fortunately BWB have anticipated this and run Cygnet Care for newcomers which, in spite of its twee name, is a first-class idea to put newcomers at their ease.

The Cygnet Care staff first of all help you decide the best route, taking your interests into account and will accompany you at the start of your trip to make sure you've got the hang of the straightforward controls for steering, starting and stopping the boat. They then explain very carefully the procedure for passing through locks — it's much simpler than you might imagine and if I can manage it anyone can. In fact some years ago a friend's ten-year-old daughter cycled most of the way through France along tow paths, handling the locks for their boat which was slowly making its way to the Mediterranean. Bicycles, incidentally, are an excellent transport back-up if you are spending a lot of time on the waterways.

A midweek break in the off season will include fuel, gas, bed linen, TV and car parking. Such a break is probably the best way to find out if waterway travel is for you. After that you could either take a longer British Waterways Leisure Trip, starting from Nantwich, or ask the appropriate BWB office to provide you with a list of hire cruiser companies in your own area.

A trip from Nantwich along the LLangollen Canal, which includes crossing the spectacular Pontcysyllte aqueduct as well as the Grindley Brook staircase locks, could turn you into a seasoned narrow boater and certainly I wouldn't dream of tackling a trip on the French waterways or buying my own boat before trying out a few journeys in Britain.

You might also try hiring a different sort of boat, say a cabin cruiser, before thinking in terms of buying your own boat which, incidentally, has no need to cost a fortune. Of course you can pay an incredible amount for boats, and big luxury yachts are generally regarded as bottomless pits into which their owners shovel money, but it's perfectly possible to pick up a sound two- to three-berth river-canal cruiser for around £1,500. If you're going to spend a lot of time on the water compare this price with the cost of staying in hotels, or renting cottages for weeks at a time, and it begins to look even more reasonable.

The best place to start looking is in the boating press, the monthly waterway magazines you can pick up at most newsagents. Once you've got an idea of the sort of thing you want — or can afford — you might try boat yards close to your home. It's quite likely that they'll have just what you want. When you've found a suitable boat it's best to have it properly vetted by a BWB recognised surveyor to check its condition, specification and value. Naturally you'll already have made sure it's narrow enough to pass through locks, but having an expert make the rest of the checks could save you expense and worry.

Insurance

There's no legal requirement to insure your boat but it certainly makes sense to do so even if you only go in for 'third party' cover. It also makes sense to cover your boat against loss and damage and to cover the safety of yourself and any crew. It really is worth it; I remember many years ago the immense pie dish in which the famous Denby Dale Pie was to be cooked sank at its moorings on the canal while on its maiden voyage from Leeds to Denby Dale. Its crew were in the pub at the time but the pie dish was insured as being A1 at Lloyds and the insurers paid out without demur.

Licensing

Once you've bought and insured your boat you do need a licence or certificate before you put in on the water and licences are based on the length of your craft.

Moorings

Unless you can get your boat out of the water and take it home on a trailer you'll need a permanent mooring approved by the BWB, details of which can be obtained from the Area Leisure Officer of BWB who can also give you information about private moorings and marinas. Surprisingly, you even need permission to moor at the end of your garden if it happens to front on a waterway but you do get a 50 per cent reduction in the fee.

For cruising the BWB provide overnight moorings in some places free of charge but they might get a bit upset if you tried to use them on a permanent basis. The waterway network has water points for taking on fresh water, refuse disposal facilities and sanitary stations where you can empty chemical loos. The BWB issue special keys for these facilities and you can obtain them from BWB offices, boat clubs and boat yards.

Houseboats

If you want to live on your boat full-time it must have a Houseboat Certificate to be moored on the waterway and, as the BWB are not keen to increase the number of these certificates, it's best to investigate your chances of getting an approved mooring before buying the boat. That being said, there are quite a number of docks and harbours not controlled by the BWB, many of which have marinas with all the facilities you would need to live aboard. The main thing is to take time to ensure that you have a place to moor your boat once it's yours.

Learning about Boats

Learning to handle a narrow boat or a canal and river cruiser won't qualify you to handle a seagoing craft, any more than flying in a balloon will enable you to fly a jet. However, it does give you the feel of being on the water and, as the speed limit on most waterways is 4 mph, or a fast walking pace, it's about as safe a way of learning about boats as you can get.

Experienced narrow boaters, for example, can obtain permission to navigate tidal waterways, which is one step nearer the open sea — if this is what you have in mind. After this you could think in terms of a cruising course at a school recognised by the RYA, many of which will undertake to train you in your own boat. If you use the school's sailing boats, which take up to a half a dozen pupils at a time, your tuition fee for the five day course will include accommodation, food and normal running expenses. Costs work out at considerably more for a power boat, although, once again, retired people can benefit from low-season reductions.

Variety

There are an incredible number of ways of getting about on water, from bath tubs to cruise liners. So far my own nautical exploits — and I'm a landlubber — include sailing in a trawler off Iceland, on a Royal Navy cruiser in the Arctic, a junk in the Pacific, a converted torpedo boat, a racing yacht in the Mediterranean and a 100 mph power boat in Bristol docks — as well as attempts at canoeing and wind surfing.

I enjoyed them all — although I could have done without some of the Arctic weather — but my latest travelling on water exploit was at 4 mph in a narrow boat and both Molly and I thought it was terrific; the peace and quiet and the totally different perspective could become addictive and we can't wait to plan another trip. In fact, though I look back on Force 9 gales and trying to drink soup with waves on it with a certain amount of nostalgia, I'm now quite prepared to sail in the comfort of a boat which is unlikely to rattle the ice in my drink.

Useful Addresses

British Waterways Board, Melbury House, Melbury Terrace, London NW1 6JX. The best source of advice for any inland waterways trip. There are several Area Leisure Offices (see Yellow Pages) and booklets, maps, advice and a news magazine are available. Information from: Leisure Division, PO Box 9, 1 Dock Street, Leeds LS1 1HH. To hire a cruiser: Hire Cruiser Booking Office, Chester Road, Nantwich CW5 8LB.

Royal Yachting Association, Victoria Way, Woking GU21 1EQ. Full membership is worth the cost — and is offered to clubs if full affiliated at a considerable discount. Booklets, advice and further discounts to members make joining well worthwhile. To join, apply to: The Membership Office, Queen Street, Gillingham SP8 4PQ

Further Reading

BWB Lockmaster Maps, British Waterways Board, London (address above). These are a series of detailed cruising maps of 26 inland waterways

BWB Sales and Hire Catalogues, British Waterways Board, London (address above). A list of all available BWB items for sale or hire including books, maps, postcards, colour slides, etc

Journey Without End, David Bolton, Methuen, London. An account of an 18-month voyage of exploration by the author and his wife through England's waterways

Narrow Boat, L.T.C. Rolt, Christopher Helm, London. A classic account of waterway travel in 1939, when the canals and inland waterways of Britain were busy commercial routes

RYA Publications List, Royal Yachting Association, Gillingham (address above). A brochure detailing practical cruising courses, clubs for newcomers, RYA activities, practical advice, etc

Self-Catering Afloat, Bill Glenton, Christopher Helm, London. Practical recipes and advice on how to eat well whilst afloat — and without too much trouble

Shell Book of Inland Waterways, Hugh McKnight, Shell Guides, London. A fascinating guide to Britain's waterways network

7

Bus, Coach and Taxi

Once upon a time local bus fares were only a couple of pennies—and real pennies at that—but what with swingeing increases in the cost of fuel and bus crews having to be paid a living wage, bus fares in many places have risen to the point where they sound more like the price of the vehicle than a ride in it. Mind you, they are still good value and perhaps seem shocking only to people like myself who have come back to buses only recently after years of using other forms of transport.

Even for regular bus travellers recent privatisation has made bus travel in many areas confusing to say the least, with—in some cases—several services instead of the familiar Corporation bus. Of course this can have advantages in popular areas with buses whizzing along every few minutes but uneconomic routes seem to have suffered and the change has meant that there are several time-tables, overlapping services and separate bus stations and enquiry offices, some of which, to make matters even more difficult, are now being phased out.

At the same time privatisation has meant that Senior Citizen concessions now vary even more than before and, in different areas of the country, range from no reductions at all to free, or virtually free, travel for the lucky ones. There have always been wide variations in concessions, some areas running a voucher system, some a fixed low rate for within a certain region and others giving a slight reduction at off-peak hours. Now, with an increase in the number of bus companies, the situation is even more confused.

If You Need Help

Fortunately there is a tremendous amount of information available if you know where to look for it and have the time to do so. When you are no longer in full-time employment it's worth the effort—especially if it's going to save money.

68

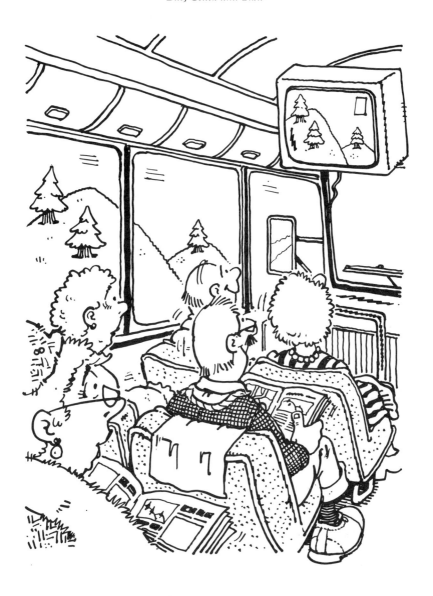

Finding one's way through the current administrative maze can even be fun as well as profitable but don't worry if you can't face a lot of 'phone calls, don't fancy quizzing a lot of people, aren't up to standing in line at an enquiry desk and can't read a time-table.

Age Concern

Help is at hand from the local branch of Age Concern. If you have difficulty coping with today's bus services explain your problem and they will advise you. They can help, too, in telling you what concessions are available, how you should go about applying for them and will often be able to suggest the best bus for a particular route. Even if you are perfectly happy to make a few 'phone calls or pop down to your nearest bus depot you could still save hassle and money by getting in touch with Age Concern in the first place.

Depending on how busy they are, and how much help you need, where they cannot give you the information themselves, they can at least save you frustration and money by telling you who to ring or where to call. This could be a big help; for instance, if you don't have a 'phone at home—feeding 10p pieces into a 'phone box, when somebody asks you to hold on and then tells you that you should have called another department on an entirely different number, is not only infuriating but expensive.

Tourist Offices

Another useful contact for bus information, especially if you are a stranger to an area, is the local tourist office where you will almost certainly find someone able to give you the information you want or tell you where to find it. Incidentally, you don't have to be a tourist to use the tourist information centre in your own town. After all, if you pay rates you are supporting it so you might just as well make use of it.

Apart from basic information about bus routes and concessions, tourist offices usually have details of a surprising number of local excursions, guided bus tours and so on that you might fancy trying now that you have the time. You could well find that you don't know your own area as well as you thought. You'll often find that the tourist office has free maps of the town centre with bus stops and places of interest marked on them. These are well worth having and fit conveniently in a pocket or handbag. They are also useful if visitors to your town stop and ask the way to somewhere; it's much easier to show them on a small map.

It's just as well to try to keep up with local changes in bus routes. Molly recently carried some heavy plants back from a garden shop over the other side of the city and then discovered that a new bus would have taken her almost door to door.

Citizens Advice Bureau

An expert on local and long distance bus travel, Ken Smith, told me recently, 'It may sound silly but the Citizens Advice Bureau is one very good place to make inquiries about local services and your Senior Citizen entitlement. There is no easy way through the maze of information, especially in a city but fortunately older people do have the time.' Ken pointed out that many older people were sometimes too shy to ask for information on concessions, perhaps because they didn't like to admit to being Senior Citizens. As someone who for a long time claimed that his daughter was adopted 'when I was very very young' rather than admit he was old enough to have a child in her twenties, I can appreciate this!

However, writing books about retirement has changed my attitude and, quite frankly, there is too much money to be saved to let vanity interefere with getting what we are entitled to.

Bus Stations
Once you've found the right bus company and the right office get all the information you need and file it for future use. Dump everything else because if there is one thing private industry produces it's lots and lots of paper.

If you want information about only one or two routes which you might be using regularly, get the bus station office staff to write down the details for you. Ask them to also give you any information about weekly, monthly or season passes, plus an application form for any concessions you may wish to apply for.

When you get home write out the details of each service—bus number, the stops where you get on and off, bus frequency or the exact time if it's a route you'll use regularly, and the price of the fare or bus pass. You could put the details of each bus route on a plain postcard using a big fat felt-tip pen. I find these sort of cards tremendously useful for everything from public speaking to shopping and they are great for writing down bus numbers and directions. They are small enough to slip in your pocket when you go out and can be kept at home in a box or drawer, perhaps in the hall.

Community Service Buses
The Citizens Advice Bureau and Age Concern can also help with information about Community Service Buses, some of which have a regular limited service to enable people without ordinary buses to get to the shops, the doctor or the dentist and so on. Some of these, depending on the district and distances, run only once or twice a week while others have a service several times a day. Age Concern even run some services themselves in certain areas. They also have information about any free trips that may be available to older people—like the one a local millionaire has offered to Bristol pensioners for many years in memory of his daughter.

Bus Shops
To help everyone—and not just pensioners—cope with the maze and to find out what is available some bus companies have set up 'Bus

Shops'. These are often located in grocers, newsagents and so on and they can be particularly helpful as you not only get advice from the shopkeeper but, in many cases, can buy your concessionary fare tickets and even Rover and Fare Cards—for regular travel between two points—direct from the shop and also get information about bargain trips.

It's worth asking about discounts for mature people even on advertised discount fares; they may not always be available but it does no harm to ask. While most age-related discounts on buses are for pensioners, it pays to ask about them if you are only over 60 and to point out that British Rail and National Express offer Senior Cards to those people of 60 who have not reached retirement age.

Hot Line

Another useful service in some areas is a Bus Company Information 'Hot Line'. This provides details of special offers along with lots of other information. Directory enquiries or, again, Age Concern should be able to get the number for you if there is one in your district.

Master Time-Tables

Some County Councils have recently realised just what a dog's breakfast their bus services seem to the lay person now that, as they put it, 'In the new era of competition, more bus companies are operating services either on their own commercial judgement or under contract.'

Avon County Council in the West Country, for example, has produced a composite time-table giving full details of all bus services in seven areas of the county which lists a total of 34 operators providing bus services in the county. These operators range from the big city boys to people running rural transport associations and taxi services. In Avon the time-tables themselves are printed in creditably clear type, but in most time-tables the typeface is bound to be pretty small so you could find a magnifying glass or one of those battery-operated map readers with a light a useful thing to keep handy.

Coach Trips and Tours in Britain

Not all coach tour operators offer reductions for Senior Citizens, but retired people can still economise by travelling outside peak holiday times which can save them between one third and one half of the cost of an inclusive 'package' of coach, hotel, excursions and so on.

Favourite destinations include seaside resorts, Scotland, the Lake District, East Anglia, Stratford and Snowdonia and the off-peak times vary according to whether the centre is used by businessmen during the week or is a favourite weekend spot.

Weatherwise, if you intend to spend much time out of the coach, walking or exploring, it could be as well to try for the 'shoulder' periods on either side of the high season. Molly took an off-peak coach tour to Scotland some time ago and hasn't stopped talking about it since—it was real value for money with centrally situated hotels, guided tours and plenty of time for looking round and—especially important for Molly's mother who went with her—the pick-up point was conveniently close to her home and, as the coach passed the house on the return journey, the driver actually dropped them off at the door.

Ken Smith's advice regarding package tours by coach is to check the small print in the brochure very carefully. 'Retired people have the time to get hold of several brochures and to compare them at leisure—in which case they'll be surprised at how expensive some of the "bargains" turn out to be. They should check, for example, if the very reasonable looking "up front" price is really inclusive or whether things like insurance, evening meals, excursions and so on are all extras. These extras can mount up dramatically so you can save yourself a lot of money by checking carefully before you book.'

What is a 'Luxury' Coach?

Coaches have improved a lot since the days of 'charas' and travellers on trips of more than a couple of hours—and often on even short journeys—can expect a high standard of comfort, a toilet, a food and drinks service and perhaps in-coach video—the latter being something of a mixed blessing unless it comes with aircraft-style individual head-sets. If not, a pair of ear plugs might be useful on a long journey.

Leg room can be a problem on cheaper tours, especially for tall people, but apart from asking about this point before you book the only thing you can do, if you are uncomfortably squashed, is to complain when you get back; of course if there are some seats which the driver knows will remain empty for the whole of a long journey a complaint to the courier or driver may lead to adjustments being made.

In Britain lack of toilet stops is rarely a problem and most drivers are friendly and caring enough, even if they appear flip and cynical. Their careworn attitude is almost certainly due to over exposure to travellers like you and me.

Motorway Problems

Incidentally, if you get off your coach at a motorway or autoroute station during the night to get a drink or call at the loo, do try to keep with other people from the coach, or at least check carefully which side of the road your coach is parked. This is particularly important when the rest station has two sections joined by a bridge and it is too dark to see your particular vehicle.

Both Molly's mother and a friend have gone into the coach park on the wrong side of an autoroute and were not very popular with other travellers when they caused a lengthy delay although they were lucky that people came to look for them. On a tour your driver or courier will check the number of passengers but it is really up to you to take care not to get lost. Even if you are tired try to make a mental note about the position of the restaurant and the toilets.

National Express

As the name implies this is a nationwide network offering scheduled services to more than 1,500 destinations in Britain—and at a very reasonable cost.

National Rapide, with daily services to more than 200 places, offers luxury coaches with reclining seats, no smoking areas, toilets, light refreshment, videos and a hostess service. There is a small supplement to pay if you travel by Rapide but it is well worth every penny.

National Express also run to Heathrow and Gatwick—usually by Rapide—and it is advisable to book in advance on these services; which applies also to overnight services to major cities from London as, at any time of the year, the National Express network is extremely popular.

Great Value

If you haven't done much coach travel before it is best to try a short journey before tackling, say, the Plymouth to Edinburgh route. However, don't be put off by thinking that a long coach trip will be too tiring. National Express offer really great value for money, especially if you are a retired person and can pick your travel times. If you are also a Senior Citizen, then you can not only take advantage of the Economy Return—which allows you to make a return journey for the price of a standard single on any day, other than Friday or Sunday—but you can also get one third off single, day return and period return fares.

In other words, you can get substantial reductions on any day of the week if you travel on coaches run by National Express. Another bit of good news is that, as far as National is concerned, whether you are a man or a woman you are a Senior Citizen within the meaning of the act when you are aged 60 and over.

Euro-line

There is a growing network of national coach services known as Euro-line. This operates from Victoria Coach Station in London and has offices in many European cities. You can often pick up these services at your local bus station — although a change may be involved when you arrive in London. Return fares are available and generally over a period valid for six months.

Reductions are not available for Senior Citizens on Irish and Continental services, but it is well worthwhile asking before you book as these regulations do change from time to time.

The Euro-line network offers a sort of 'halfway' stage between the organised package tour and the local bus service. Of course, many older people will find the security of an organised package tour reassuring, where everything is organised in advance, there are helpful couriers, refreshment stops and, above all, no language difficulties. Many people won't wish to try anything more adventurous and if you're not very nimble on your feet you won't want to be hopping on and off local transport. However, if you fancy an independent trip you could try Euro-line with perhaps a few side trips on local buses. Hal Newell, for example, who has travelled all over the world, uses local transport whenever possible and finds it a great deal cheaper than organised excursions. And as a solo traveller he enjoys mixing with the locals wherever he goes.

European Travel

Using local transport for short journeys once you have established a base at your hotel, apartment or caravan, is good fun as well as being cheap and, as Hal says, it's a great way to meet the natives. Once you've had a baby plonked on your knee by a smiling mother encumbered by two other small children or have been firmly wedged into your seat by piled high market baskets you'll know you are abroad — and can settle down to enjoy it. As Ken points out, it all depends on whether you want to travel in a sort of British capsule — which many people enjoy — or whether you want to get to know the people of the country you are visiting.

Check with the local tourist office where you are staying. They can advise you about scheduled services, time-tables, special trips to places of interest and so on. There is almost always someone who can speak English — in most larger offices all the staff speak English — so don't forget to ask if there are concessions for Senior Citizens.

Seat-only Deals

If you want to visit relatives or friends who live in a remote spot which attracts coach tours, it is worth checking to see if you can get a 'seat-only' deal from a coach tour operator. It may not work, but it is worth a try as the operator would rather fill a seat than leave it empty. Try your travel agent too, he will know of cheap or bargain coach deals along these lines.

Seat-only is one way also in which you can travel independently in Europe and still have the advantages of a package tour. By travelling out with a tour group you could, for example, find a seat-only vacancy on a day trip to Paris. You can then arrange with the operator a fixed date and time to be picked up for the return journey on his next trip. This is quite feasible with a friendly operator or travel agent—although the cost of Euro-line scheduled services is now so reasonable it might not be worth it for somewhere as popular as Paris. On the other hand, if you wanted to spend some time in Klein Kleckersdorf, or some other place off the beaten track—but featured as a tourist spot—it could be worth talking to your travel agent about the seat-only option.

Happy Buses—Magic Buses

If you put peace of mind before economy it's worth paying a few pounds extra to ensure that you have a coach with an English-speaking driver who is working for a British company; otherwise you could find yourself on a descendant of the legendary Happy Bus or Magic Bus. Generally speaking, foreign coaches and their drivers have improved a lot during the last couple of years but there are still some head bangers around who will happily demonstrate, for instance, how to change drivers on the autoroute without bothering to stop the coach.

The Magic Bus—usually a double decker—used to run to Spain and although it tended to be a bit hairy at times it had a nice mixture of students and sun-seeking pensioners and was nothing like the Happy Bus. Some time ago our daughter travelled to Greece on what must have been one of the originals with kamikaze drunken drivers who were determined to complete the journey in the shortest possible time. This entailed refusing to stop anywhere other than was absolutely necessary, which in the days before on-board toilets was rarely enough and, even at her age, she wouldn't want to repeat the experience.

More recently I went to Spain on an El Cheapo coach trip and had a horrendous outward journey because the French driver hadn't heard of toilet stops and was only persuaded to pull up when we told him that if he didn't get us to a loo quickly we were going to use his shoes instead!

The redoubtable Hal Newell recalls a trip on the Happy Bus which reached a mountain village in Greece where the driver was told to take on board an elderly man who had been injured in a hit and run accident and deliver him to the hospital further up the mountain. While the arguments were going on the man stopped breathing but the Mayor insisted that he be delivered nonetheless to the hospital so he was bundled into the aisle with scant ceremony and the bus set off. To Hal's astonishment, as the bus bumped over the rocky track the 'corpse' sat up with a groan to which no one paid any attention. Two more relapses and resuscitations later the man was helped off the bus looking not much the worse for wear! As Hal says, 'It was a hell of a way to get a free ride!' but not many people would want to go that far.

The worst of the rogue companies seem to have been weeded out — although it pays to check carefully before you book — but there is still a lot of cheap coach travel to be had. Watch out for bargains in your local paper by all means — the free sheets are often a particularly good source of bargain coach travel — but unless you know the reputation of the operator offering the bargain it's best to ask around to make sure he's not going to hand you over to the mercies of some Continental cowboy. This is where you can consult your travel agent. Mention the name to him; he may not recommend the operators — he may even suggest an alternative — but he won't condemn them unless he's sure of his facts. If he does — avoid them. It's not worth the risk.

Day Trips

Apart from being a possible mode of cheap seat-only travel, day trips can be fun. The Continental Hypermarket bargains are well worth having, but the long distances and the lack of sleep can be tiring, especially if you are not used to coach travel. However many of these bargains are arranged by clubs and Senior Citizen groups, or by local newspapers catering for mixed ages, and anyone we know who has tried these has had a great time.

Clubs are also useful for 'special interest' trips and Molly's mother used to love a coach visit up to Lancashire to visit a mill warehouse where great bargains could be had in loom ends of cotton, wool and so on. The trip was arranged by a club secretary and included an arranged stop for lunch and tea and biscuits at the factory.

Comfort

Whichever type of long-distance coach travel you decide on, loose comfortable clothing is essential. Shoes should be loose fitting — I wear the zipped slip-on type that I can unfasten completely, which is bliss, and still fasten in a hurry if need be. Don't wear a tight belt or anything with tight sleeves as they will constrict your body and cause numbness in your arms and legs.

77

Do take advantage of every stop to stretch your legs and get some fresh air, whether you want refreshment or not. If you know you are prone to cramp when you sit in one position for a long time try to remember to take a cramp tablet the night before and keep one in your pocket or handbag—and if you do get cramp stand up immediately.

Most coaches allow for at least one large suitcase per person—check with your travel agent if you know you will need more although it's best to manage if you can. Molly's mother, Edith, and Aunt Alice paid for extra cases on one occasion when they went to Spain for several months but had to put up with scowls when the coach broke down and they were unable to deal with all their own luggage. They did get help from a young boy but decided that in future they would cut down on the amount they took. After that Edith limited herself to a Fido-type suitcase on wheels that she could pull on a short lead, plus a lightweight shoulder bag. The lightweight bag that you can take on as hand luggage is a must and could perhaps include disposable face cleaners, a few sweets, a change of tights or socks and perhaps a small thermos of tea or cold juice. Coaches can suffer mechanical failure or get caught in traffic jams so I usually take a medium weight pullover and a cagoule to cope with any changes in temperature or the weather *en route*. You could get soaked merely dashing for a pub or a motorway restaurant—even if you are up to dashing.

I've usually used my pullover as a makeshift pillow but Molly's mother had a much better idea which Molly still uses. This is the small, shaped neck-pillow which turns a cold hard window into a comfortable headrest and enables you to get a good night's sleep without waking up with a neck that feels as though Big Daddy has had it in a headlock. It really is a first-class idea and it has survived countless journeys mainly because of the press studded strap my mother-in-law fitted so that she could wear it on her arm or fasten it to the handle of her suitcase when on the move. It certainly gave the other passengers something to talk about and of course that's one good thing about coach travel—retired or not—it gives you more topics of conversation than almost any other form of transport.

Taxis

Wherever you may be—at home or abroad—taxis are an option well worth considering for the older traveller and, even if economy is a consideration, a short ride in a taxi can be a boon when you are feeling a bit tired or your feet aren't too good. Drivers are usually helpful to older people, especially if you have luggage, and they are often a useful source of information in a strange town or country.

Costs vary tremendously—in Britain we've found Liverpool and

Edinburgh surprisingly cheap, with cheerful considerate drivers — but generally prices won't break the bank, especially if there are two or more of you travelling, in which case it can sometimes be as cheap as public transport. Taxis — originally 'taxi-meter cabriolets' — should have meters, so you can see how much you should pay per unit of distance, adding a specified amount for luggage and extra passengers. If the cab has no meter it's best to fix a fare before getting in and don't be afraid to haggle.

This is especially important at airports which are invariably sited in the next county to where you want to be and where some of the cabs should definitely be flying the Jolly Roger. Retired travellers like us could do well to leave airport taxis to the expense account flyers and check on the availability of airport buses, hotel or travel firm courtesy cars or public transport. This is where a limited amount of luggage — say, one case with wheels and a shoulder bag — gives you much more freedom of choice than if you are lugging round even three things.

If you really do have to use a taxi after all then ask at the airport information desk what the going rate is and approximately how far it is to your destination. Better still — when you are coming in to land — you might ask anyone sitting near you in the aircraft about local taxis. Who knows, you could be invited to share a cab or for that matter be offered a lift in a Rolls!

Useful Addresses

Age Concern, Bernard Sunley House, 60 Pitcairn Road, Mitcham, London
   CR4 3LL. Telephone (01) 640 5431
Citizens Advice Bureau, local telephone directory

8

Railways — They're Getting You There!

Archie Macfarlane is 89-years-old. He gets a lot of use out of his Senior Citizen Railcard because he uses it to travel up to Hereford from his home near Bristol to go free-fall parachuting with men from the Special Air Service (SAS). Archie, who took up parachuting when he was 75 and has now been retired from his job as an aircraft fitter with Rolls-Royce for a quarter of a century, also uses his Railcard to help him in his other hobby — mountain climbing — and since he sold his motorbike and colour TV to finance a trip to see his son in Rhodesia he finds the train both convenient and cheap.

Travelling at weekends on his Railcard he can get up to Hereford for about £5 for a day return, which is not only good value but in his case has a positive advantage over motor-cycling. Said Archie, 'The SAS are a great bunch of lads but they are a bit wild and if there's no jumping we get into the pub and I find it difficult to say "No" to a drink.'

Unsurprisingly, Archie was adopted as a mascot by the British Rail (BR) team when they ran a competition in which Railcard holders were offered a chance to win their 'Trip of a Lifetime'; they took just one look at his application before deciding to award him his particular 'experience' by taking him out for a day's stunt-flying.

Of course not all of us care to go parachuting, stunt-flying or even the sort of mountain scrambling that Archie still enjoys, but he has been travelling in retirement for longer than most of us so his advice is worth listening to. Mind you I have to confess that as the son and grandson of railwaymen I am predisposed in favour of railways and have marvellous memories of boyhood rail journeys from one end of the country to the other. Those were the days when first-class carriages had armchair comfort, a bell to ring for attendance and often their own loos and washbasins. Meals in the first-class dining car were protracted affairs of four or five courses with spotless white napery and gleaming cutlery. Regal travel indeed, but it wasn't available to all

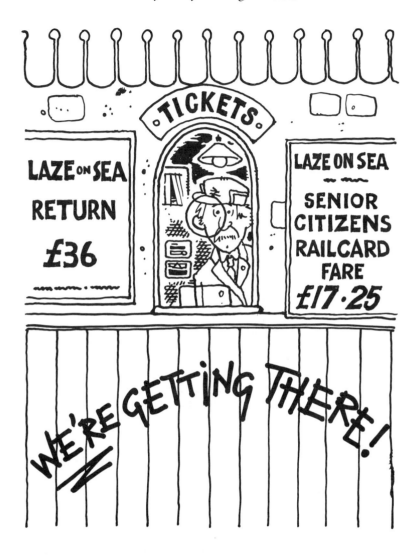

and, having been spoiled rotten, I was surprised on occasions to encounter such joys as dirty non-corridor rolling stock, ice-cold carriages with torn seats and engines that performed with markedly less reliability than those pulling the Pines Express or the Flying Scotsman of the old days.

Harking back to the 'good old days' of rail travel is fine as long as we remember that, as in most things, our memories of pre-Beeching railways tend to be selective. Indeed our railway memories in general

81

tend to be more rose coloured than others, if only because so many of us still find steam trains romantic and forget that they were often smoky and smelly.

Molly and I did a great deal of rail travel recently when we were publicising our book *Cooking in Retirement*. Although we got well off our regular routes we found rail travel extremely comfortable and convenient. Not only that, but the ancillary services that used to be something of a joke after they were run down so badly in the Second World War are now a lot better, even if they are largely geared to self-service. Of course buffets do leave a lot to be desired when compared with those first-class dining cars of old but you can't have everything —and besides, there's nothing to stop us taking a leaf out of the really old-fashioned railway traveller's book and putting up a splendid picnic basket.

The only thing really wrong with rail travel in Britain today is the horrendous price of a ticket; in fact if you have to travel frequently or cover long distances you almost have to mortgage your house— unless, that is, you happen to be retired and over 60. Like all transport concerns, BR are prepared to go to great lengths to fill seats which would otherwise remain empty at off-peak periods and in this respect their problem is greater than that of their competitors as they aren't really able to go in for a lot of fancy re-scheduling. There is still an element of public service in the railway system, which means that BR must often run trains even if there are hardly any passengers— although of course they would much rather not. To get bottoms on seats they offer some very attractive deals but the snag is that—at least at first sight—it seems that to take advantage of them you have to be a registered Zoroastrian, non-smoking, one-legged, flute player travelling after 11.30 a.m. on a Thursday in the second week after Michaelmas.

Like many other retired people who travel by train Archie Macfarlane has found out how to get the best out of a system which isn't quite as complicated as it looks. He does this in two ways, depending on what sort of travel he's doing and whether it involves a set destination or is purely recreational when he just wants a cheap and interesting day out.

In both cases he goes down to his local Travel Centre at Bristol Temple Meads Station and gets his information not only direct from the horse's mouth but at his leisure. 'I go down there a couple of days before I want to go off anywhere and they tell me if there are any good bargains coming up to that particular destination. At the same time I find out if there are any interesting special trips or deals on offer. I also keep my eye open for advertisements of special offers in the local papers but you can't really beat going to the station.

'Travelling by train,' he added, 'especially from main line stations is much easier these days than it used to be, thanks to the electronic notice boards that tell you exactly what is happening and which platform a train's arriving at.'

In many ways I prefer the human touch and still tend to ask a railman to confirm the information displayed on the screen but, having once boarded a train for Denmark at Hamburg Main Railway Station when I really wanted to go to Holland, I can see that the modern system does have its advantages.

What's on Offer

Philip Bradford, British Rail Travel Centre Manager, confirmed that Archie has the right formula for retirement rail travel. 'Retired travellers are ideally suited to get the best deal from us,' Philip said, 'not only because they are able to travel at cheap off-peak times but they also have the leisure to plan their journeys ahead and to make their enquiries and bookings in advance, changing perhaps to another day if there's a special offer coming up. Of course to take advantage of all the services we offer it's almost always better—and in some cases absolutely essential—to have everything fixed up beforehand. Our booking office staff are highly trained and they know all about reduced fares, special offers and so on but if you arrive at the ticket window two minutes before the train is due and there's a long queue of travellers waiting to buy tickets it's difficult for them to spare the time to tell you all about the best and cheapest way to travel. In other words, you could miss out on a money-saving fare if you don't take the time to visit or at least phone your local Travel Centre.'

Incidentally, visiting a mainline Travel Centre is now a lot more comfortable than standing in front of an 'Enquiries' window. Most of them have comfortable armchairs to sit on while you browse through the various brochures and pamphlets detailing current BR offers and the staff no longer look at you pityingly if you confess to being baffled by the time-tables or unable to read the small print. Of course, being helpful and friendly is part of their job but I like to think that my father and my grandfather—both of whom would have spoken severely to anyone they thought was being churlish to passengers—would welcome this return to one of the things that was really good about railways in the 'good old days'.

Life begins at 60 with a Senior Citizen Railcard
If you are no longer in full-time employment you are well placed to find out about and enjoy the best of travel bargains offered to ordinary passengers; but for retired people who like to travel by rail life really does begin at 60. As soon as you reach the magic 60 you are eligible

for a Senior Citizen Railcard—the card that British Rail refer to as 'a passport to cheaper rail travel'. The only snag, as far as I can see, is that you—sorry, we—have to admit to being over 60, which is a bit rough if you've been claiming a 'footballing age' of a few years less; but think of the money you'll save!

More seriously, it's as well to remember when you are thinking of buying a Railcard that no suspicion of charity attaches to the scheme because, although BR have become a little more service-orientated than they were some years ago, they are still by no means altruistic and the whole purpose of the exercise is to fill seats. That being said, it's still a brilliant deal if you make full use of your card.

To get hold of a card first check if you are eligible—in other words, over 60 and a British resident, or over 60, of British nationality and living outside Britain. You can buy a Railcard at most major BR stations, at Post Offices and at Rail Appointed Travel Agents but—especially if you look young and beautiful—you are going to have to prove you really are who and what you claim.

You can do this with:

(1) Your pension book or any DHSS document which proves you are eligible for a state retirement pension
(2) Your passport or a NHS medical card confirming your date of birth *plus* a postmarked letter such as a gas or electricity bill confirming you are a *bona fide* British resident
(3) Your birth certificate *plus* a postmarked letter addressed to you personally

You'll be pleased to know that this is a once only procedure and that producing your previous Senior Citizen Railcard is all you need to do when getting a subsequent one.

The application form is simple and there is one question asking about your interests or hobbies which—provided you don't tick a box to request otherwise—should ensure that you get a steady stream of travel offers and information, much of which will relate to your special interests.

With the card you get one third off Saver Tickets. This is brilliant because it's available for most Second Class journeys over 50 miles or so. You travel outward on the day shown and return within a month. There are, however, a few restrictions on trains to and from or via London so if the capital is on your route it pays to consult your Travel Centre before booking.

A Senior Citizen Railcard will also entitle you to 34 per cent off a Rail Rover Ticket—which is good value in the first place as it offers unlimited travel during a specific period for a set sum.

Card holders can purchase reduced price Underground tickets

after 9.30 am Monday to Friday and all day at weekends and Public Holidays.

If there isn't an available Saver or Day Return you can still save money by getting one third off ordinary singles—a facility which is also valid for First Class travel. This enables you to travel at any time and is useful if you have to travel when Savers or Cheap Day Returns aren't available. There's also one third off Standard Returns—both First and Second Class—for journeys over 30 miles, travelling at any time and returning within three months.

Enjoy your journey without worrying about getting a seat. A Second Class seat reservation costs just £1 each way and First Class £2, and if you are travelling as a group you can get four reservations together in Second Class for £1 each way.

Travelling First Class

Retired people who have been used to travelling by train on an expense account are in for a rude shock when they have to pay for their own tickets as I discovered when, after years of luxury train travel—courtesy of my father and my employers—I found myself on my own. As I recall, I underwent a Road to Damascus style sudden conversion to democracy on the move and Second Class tickets—the only exception being an occasional business trip where I was able to claw back some of the money, or times when I needed the confidence-boosting aura of First Class travel.

As Philip Bradford pointed out, if you are travelling at the week-end—when the expense account brigade rarely use the trains—you can go First Class on payment of a small supplement. This means that if you are using your Railcard to travel at reduced weekend rates, which gives you a double discount on Second Class Fares, you can gild the lily for a few pounds and travel First Class. For an older person, particularly on long journeys, this can be a real boon. Incidentally, you can take up to four children under 16 at a set price per head (currently £1) whenever you go, except when travelling first class.

Whether you want to travel First or Second, getting the most out of your Senior Citizen Railcard is something of a game and the people most likely to know all the rules—and the up to the minute rules at that—are the staff at your nearest Travel Centre. One way they can make life easier, as well as cheaper, for older folk is in helping them reserve seats, which is not very costly and in some cases is absolutely free. Naturally you have to reserve your seat before you travel but it is well worth it to avoid having to stand or sit on your case from London to Glasgow.

Incidentally, if you do find you are in a really full train don't be shy about asking, 'Is this seat taken?'. It is worth asking as otherwise you could be standing while someone else's parcel has a comfortable seat, just to give its selfish owner a bit more elbow or leg room. If this doesn't work, try the buffet car or the bar. The rule, by the way, is that your ticket entitles you to transport and not a seat, unless you have reserved one. However if you have paid for First Class and are forced to travel Standard—as BR now call Second Class—you can claim a refund of the difference.

Train Travel for the Disabled

Though not an altruistic organisation—they are, after all, in the business to make money—BR do, in the case of rail travel for the frail and disabled, offer a remarkable service on which they almost certainly lose money.

For instance, in these days when most porters no longer port, they can arrange for you to have assistance with heavy luggage if you are elderly, frail—or even if you happen to have hurt your back—and this can range from provision of a BR trolley to a full portering service including help in changing trains where appropriate. Obviously, if more than a trolley is required you have to notify BR of your needs well in advance and in most Travel Centres there is now a specially trained member of staff to deal with people who need extra help of this sort.

For the more severely disabled, BR wheelchairs are available and if you have your own wheelchair and are unable to travel in an ordinary seat the Travel Centre will arrange for you to be met outside the station and taken to a First Class carriage where a seat has been removed to accommodate a wheelchair. They will also telephone your destination—or, in the case of changes, the inter-mediate stations—to arrange help with transfers. This service won't cost you anything above Standard rate and your escort can also travel in the seat opposite yours at Standard rate.

Train Travel in Europe

For Senior Citizen Railcard holders there are some great bargains to be had in European travel. If you already have a Senior Citizen Railcard, the Rail Europ Senior card costs only £5 and reductions are available on single, return or circular journeys, either First or Standard class, and are based on full price ordinary fares.

You can save up to half the fare on railways in Belgium, France,

Finland, Greece, Luxembourg, the Netherlands, Norway, Portugal, the Republic of Ireland, Spain, Sweden and most Swiss Railways. You can also get up to 30 per cent off fares on railways in Austria, Denmark, West Germany and Italy, as well as behind the Iron Curtain in Hungary and Yugoslavia.

In addition, you save up to half the fare on BR when you buy a through-international—rail-sea ticket and up to 30 per cent on sea crossings to the Continent by Sealink, Hoverspeed and Townsend Thoresen services between Dover and Ostend or between Portsmouth and Le Havre—when these are part of a rail-sea journey.

As a Senior Citizen with a Rail Europ Senior Card, for example, you can get to Paris for under £25 return or as far as Cannes for under £50—which can't be bad. There is no reduction for *Frances Vacances*—the French equivalent of Rail Rover—but for about £50 you can travel anywhere in France on any four days during a period of 15 days and for about £100 on any nine days during a one month period.

People like Hal Newell don't go for Rail Rovers a lot because they think it cuts out the element of happenstance and means they would have wasted their money if someone offers them a free lift, but given the 15 days in which to take advantage of the card I'll take my chance and if someone offers me a free trip or a cruise or something equally tempting before I've had the chance to use up my Railcard days I'm not going to cry too much. On Birmingham New Street station recently we met an elderly New Zealand couple who had worked out that they just had time to nip down to have a look at Bath before their card expired. They had quickly become experts on time-tables, had found everyone very helpful and had visited friends and relatives all over the place.

If you like the idea of package holidays but don't fancy being a package—especially among hordes of noisy juvenile packages—Golden Rail Holidays, a subsidiary of BR, offer a wide range of holidays in Britain and Europe, from one night upwards, which are specifically designed for the over-55s. They are a bit up-market and not particularly cheap but they do offer value for money plus the company of people in a similar age group to oneself. They often combine a full package of rail journeys—and sea or air travel where appropriate—with rooms with private facilities and usually breakfast and dinner each day, plus a couple of coach tours included in the price. All of them offer some form of saving to holders of Senior Citizen Railcards and there are also reductions for the off season of which retired people can take full advantage. Seven nights in Dunoon, for example, including one full day and two half-day trips costs from well under £150 off season with reductions for Railcard holders. Not too bad for featherbed travel and accommodation, and you can travel First Class for an extra 10 per cent or so; in fact it's probably better than you could fix up yourself and that's always the acid test for package travel.

As always, the best thing is to ask for the latest information about reductions for older travellers as things tend to change from year to year. Ask British Rail Travel Centres, especially at Victoria, any ABTA travel agent—Thomas Cook is particularly good—or the London Office of the Rail System concerned.

Austria

Austria offers 30 per cent off standard fares if you have a Rail Europ Card. However, if you buy their special Senior Citizen's card you can get 50 per cent off, so if you are over 60 a lot depends on how good your arithmetic is and how much rail travelling you intend to do in Austria.

Foreign visitors, no matter what their age, can get an 'Austrian Ticket' which is like BR's Rail Rover but can be used not only on Austrian trains but on Railway and Post Office buses, the Vienna Schnellbahn system, the steamers on the Wolfgangsee and even some cog railways. In addition the tickets also provide a 50 per cent reduction on scheduled lines on the Danube and the Bodensee—which means that over a period, say, of nine days you could soon get your money's worth.

France

The *Carte Vermeille* is now only available to French citizens but you can save up to 50 per cent on French railways if you have a Rail Europ Card. For the under-60s there are the *Cartes Vacances* at £50 for 4 days travel within a 15 day period, £105 for 9 days within a month and £130 for 16 separate days. These cards also give you Metro concessions, a 50 per cent reduction on Hoverspeed plus discounts from some hotels. If you intend doing a fair amount of train travel and have a good idea of where you want to go—and when—this can be a money saver, but unless you are a Senior Wrangler it's a good idea to plan your journeys in detail and then consult either BR or the SNCF French Railways office in London well in advance.

Germany

If you enjoy lots of train travel you'll find the Bundesbahn runs more than 20,000 passenger trains a day with a splendid Intercity network covering 50 cities. Trains run at hourly intervals and you can save 30 per cent with a Rail Europ Card.

The Deutsche Bundesbahn Tourist Card costs £55 for four days, £82 for nine days and £113 for 16 days of unlimited travel and is valid on Rhine and Rhine/Moselle Line coaches and some steamers so, once again, it's a question of how much travelling you intend to do. If you are really flush and intend making train travel a big feature of your trip they also do a First-Class Tourist Card.

Holland

With a Rail Europ Card there's 50 per cent off and there are cheap returns or tourist tickets if you intend travelling a lot. The Dutch have one of the best rail services in the world—comfortable, frequent and dependable. Rail Rover tickets valid for 3 to 7 days and offering unlimited travel have a Link option giving unlimited travel on public transport in all the big cities.

Italy

There is a good rail network covering the whole of Italy. Fares are reasonable and there is up to 30 per cent off for holders of Rail Europ Senior Cards. However, whatever influence the late Signor Mussolini may have had on rail punctuality seems to have been dissipated, especially at local train level. The best—and the most expensive—are the Super Rapide trains which have only First Class seats and on which reservations are essential.

If you intend doing a lot of travel by rail the Travel at Will tickets for 8, 15, 21 or 30 days can be good value. Between main stations the 'expresso' is almost an express, stopping only at main line stations, but the 'rapido' is even better, although you do need a reservation and often have to pay a supplement as well. One unusual option is the 'Chilmetrico' which offers 3,000 kilometres for 90,000 Lira Second Class or 160,000 Lira First Class and can be used by up to five people at the same time for a maximum of 20 journeys. Interesting if you can figure out the odds but I gave up trying to work out these sort of problems on the day I scraped through School Certificate maths. If you don't have a Rail Europ Card and are only going to make the occasional train journey the Circular Returns which enable you to travel out by one route and come back by another could be interesting, although not particularly economical, and there are also Tourist discounts on day and three-day returns.

Spain

The Spanish National Railways offer savings of up to 50 per cent to holders of Rail Europ Senior Citizen Cards and there are Tourist Cards available at £50 for 8 days of travel, but it has to be said that the Spanish rail service is not the best in the world.

The best trains are the Telgo and Ter services but you have to pay a supplement to travel on these. The 'expresso' and 'rapido' trains seem to have been named on the 'wishing will make it so' principle, while the 'tranvia', 'correo' and 'ferobus' are frequently interesting exercises in Mañana-motion. In fact, apart from the crack trains mentioned above, rail travel in Spain should perhaps be regarded as more of an experience than a means of getting from one place to another.

Romancing the Rail

There is still something romantic about rail travel, especially for people who remember the age of steam, perhaps because the mere sound of a steam whistle brings back memories of childhood holidays and the meetings and partings that made trains such a part of our lives when not all of us had cars. One of my all-time thrills, for example, was to drive a steam locomotive between Newcastle and Crewe and another was to drive a replica of Stephenson's Rocket and I still find travelling by any sort of train romantic.

The trouble with this particular romance is that, like most romances, it can be expensive and it's just as well that retired people have the time to find out how best to make the fares structure work for them—whether they are going free-fall parachuting like Archie Macfarlane or taking their grandchildren for a day out. In fact, once you've cracked the system—and it's just a question of geting the best possible advice—rail travel can be travel in retirement at its best.

Useful Addresses

DER Travel Service, 18 Conduit Street, London. Telephone (01) 408 0111. Details on rail travel throughout Germany

SNCF French Railways Limited, 179 Piccadilly, London. Telephone (01) 439 9927

Further Reading

ABC Rail Guide, ABC Travel Guides, Dunstable. Monthly publication of up-to-date rail travel information

British Rail Leaflets. There are many of these, most available from your local railway station, some travel agents, etc. Specialist ones include *Travelling with British Rail*—a guide for disabled people. Invaluable station-by-station details such as facilities for parking, level access, toilets, availability of wheelchairs. Has telephone numbers disabled people can check ahead with when planning trip. *Golden Rail Holidays*—for the over 55s. *Rail Europ Senior Card* leaflet and *Senior Citizen Rail Card* leaflet

Going Alone (The Woman's Guide to Travel Know-how), Carole Chester, Christopher Helm, London

Holidays, Greater London Association for Pre-Retirement, London. This booklet lists those concessions available in various European countries. Obtainable only from the Association offices: St Margaret Pattens Church, Eastcheap, London EC3M 1HS

Steaming Through Britain, Anthony Burton, Deutsch, London. A railway enthusiast's guide to preserved steam railways

Thomas Cook Railpass Guide, Thomas Cook Timetable Publishing Office, PO Box 36, Peterborough PE3 6SB. Detailed information on rover tickets and railpasses for the whole of Europe plus up to date information on the rest of the world

Your Holidays, Age Concern, Bernard Sunley House, 60 Pitcairn Road, Mitcham, London CR4 3LL. Telephone (01) 640 5431

9

Up, Up and Away!

Once upon a time, when newspapers were in the business of granting wishes Jimmy Saville style, I spent so much time in the air reporting on older people who wanted to make their very first flight that it would have paid the newspaper to buy its own aircraft.

Nowadays almost every pensioner has put in more flying hours than Lindberg and they all seem to enjoy it hugely, but there must be some older people who have not yet flown and who may be a little apprehensive about leaving the ground. If you're one of them, you have my sympathy, as I've always been something of a white knuckle flyer myself—less so since I've flown in gliders, balloons and light aircraft, but I still have to remind myself that flying is statistically safer than any other mode of travel and that I am much more likely to be hurt crossing the road than in the air.

For older people who are a bit worried about flying, a 'joyride' from their local airfield could be the answer, but in fact airlines nowadays control the in-flight environment to such an extent that unless, like me, you enjoy looking out of the window, you will hardly know that you are in the air at all. Not only that, but most of us today are so used to watching people on TV flying all over the place—not to mention hearing our friends boast about their air travel— that we regard flying as a matter of course. In many ways this is a pity because apart from being quick and convenient it is a miraculous experience in its own right. If you've never skimmed low over the sea or the Finnish lakes or seen a carpet of cloud beneath the wings looking solid enough to walk on and stretching to infinity you have the experience of a lifetime ahead of you.

Airports

Getting to the airport and boarding the aircraft can be much more nerve wracking than most flying but in this respect flying in retirement

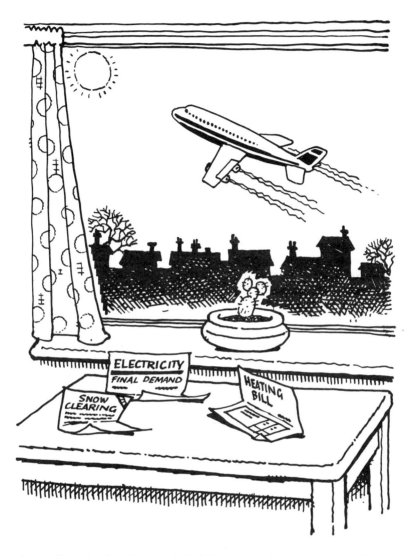

is usually easier than for people in full-time work who have to stick to a tight schedule.

For one thing we usually have more time to plan the whole exercise from the packing stage onward, which means that we have worked out in advance how we are going to get to the airport, which part of it we need—if we are flying from a big international airport like Heathrow or Gatwick—and, if we are driving ourselves, where we are going to park the car.

Smaller airports like Bristol, are friendly human-scale operations where, at certain times of the year, you can even park your car for free. Their compact size with everything close to hand makes them ideal for the older first time air traveller, especially now that you can make long-distance flights via places like Schipol.

Places like Heathrow, on the other hand, can seem a little daunting because of their size but this is only a first impression and, although it is a huge place, I have always found the staff there helpful and kind, especially if I am having one of my occasional White Rabbit attacks of the dithers.

Time to Spare

When travelling by air—and especially from places like Heathrow—retired travellers have one major advantage that we've mentioned before in that they can usually get to the airport with plenty of time to spare. This is really important as arriving at the last minute is stressful enough for a young executive and is something that older people should avoid. If your family or friends are taking you to the airport do let them know that you want to arrive particularly early—even if you have to make a joke about always being an hour early for everything. If you are travelling by coach or tube or airport bus, try to get one that leaves you plenty of time and of course if you are taking your car to the airport try to plan accordingly. It's much better to have a quiet drink and start your trip feeling relaxed than start off flustered and wondering if you've forgotten something vital.

Check-In

Printed inside your ticket you will usually find your check-in time—although in some cases you may just be told the details when you book your flight—in any case this is vital information as is your flight number. I like to write my check-in time, my flight number and the name of the airline on one of my memory postcards in letters big enough to read easily so that I have them on hand in my pocket. The check-in time is the latest time that the airline will allow you to reach their desk in order to complete the formalities connected with baggage, customs, seating and so on. Arriving much earlier than the last check-in time makes sense for older people because it means you can be dealt with before the queues start to form and it reduces your chances of being 'bumped' or losing your seat because of over-booking. Overbooking, incidentally, is the airline's defence mechanism against 'no-shows'—mainly business people who book themselves onto two or three flights to make sure of a seat—and it's surprising that the guessing game works out as well as it usually does. Still, if you arrive early you should avoid any chance of guesswork with *your* seat.

Airport Lounges

Airports are fascinating places—especially the huge ones like Heathrow and Gatwick which have everything from a medical centre (great if you have forgotten your jabs or, as I once did, get raging toothache between flights) to translators. *The Complete Sky Traveller* is a book worth consulting as it has maps of most British airports which give a good general impression of them, but only *visiting* a major airport can give you any idea of what they are really like. In fact, if you live close to an airport of any kind it's well worth visiting as a spectator before you travel and, if you can, try to make the visit in the company of an experienced air traveller. That way you will feel quite at home when you arrive for your trip and will be able to identify the check-in counter, the information desk, the bureau de change (although you'll already have what foreign cash you need with you) the restaurants, the rendezvous points, the chapel, the shops—and, of course, the toilets. You'll also have realised by this time that what makes international airports so fascinating is the people and you'll probably have started playing the never-ending game of trying to guess whether the sophisticated traveller sitting next to you in the waiting area is flying off to Bangladesh or Benidorm and, if you're not mistaken, didn't you see her on TV last week in that American comedy? She's probably wondering the same about you.

Of course, if you are flying as part of a package tour most of the planning is done for you, which gives you time to sit and stare—no bad thing as it will help you to relax before your flight. Even so, it is as well to write down the details of your flight, plus the name and telephone number of your tour company on a postcard—just in case you do get lost, either at the airport or on the way to it.

Even if you are going on an organised trip it is still a good idea to allow yourself some extra time and to use it to check things out for when eventually you do decide to go solo. If you know where everything is and how it works you will feel more comfortable. Also, in the event of a delay, if you have packed a small amount of food and drink carried for just such an emergency, you can sit quietly and plan your next move while everyone else dashes about. You have the time to relax.

In the Aircraft

It is a peculiar thing about airports that almost everyone you see looks like an experienced not to say blasé traveller but the truth is that well over two thirds of the world's population have never flown at all and everyone, almost without exception, has one or two butterflies before take off.

I normally have a complete lepidoptery collection and have been known to drown the little blighters but this is not advisable. One stiff drink is okay—a short rather than a beer for obvious reasons—but excitement and altitude cause alcohol to have more effect than usual and it wouldn't do for people of our age to be refused permission to board or to be keel-hauled for raucous singing! If you do think you may have real trouble with your nerves you could ask your doctor to prescribe a tranquilliser although most people find that butterflies vanish as if by magic once the aircraft is up and cruising.

If you are still worried, hesitating about an overseas visit because of it, it might be better to try a short internal flight—the flip around the local airfield again—before taking off to visit relatives in Australia or Canada. Or, try a British Airways 'happy hour' flight from Manchester and Birmingham. But, in most cases, once you are up in the air you'll find that not only are you able to relax and enjoy one of modern life's miracles but that, curiously enough, you have left most of your minor worries on the ground.

When you board the aircraft, try to remember your seat number and whether you've opted for smoking or non-smoking and aisle or window seat but don't worry. Cabin staff are chosen for their unruffled calm and provided you hang onto your boarding pass—*a must*—they'll make sure you reach your seat safely.

It doesn't matter if you sit on the ends of your seat belt and have to ferret round for them—it's all part of the cabaret and other people are too busy worrying about their own seat belts to notice. I've even been known to sit on the ends of my neighbour's seat belt—which at least breaks the ice. In fact as nearly everyone behaves with the suave grace of a Monsieur Hulot, especially in the crowded conditions of a charter flight, there isn't usually much ice left to break after take off and in many cases lifelong friendships are struck up which last at least until the aircraft comes to rest after landing.

Naturally you'll be wearing loose comfortable clothing—especially shoes—because people get bigger on planes and it's essential to feel at ease. Then all you have to do is to watch the cabin staff demonstrating how to wear a lifejacket and so on, check the position of the emergency exits and then lean back and wait for someone to bring you a drink—soft or otherwise. If you are anything like me, by the time you've got your shoes loosened and a large G and T in your hand you'll be convinced that flying is the only way to travel. Incidentally, don't worry about changes in the engine noise; these may be a bit disconcerting but are as normal as the noises a car's engine makes when the driver changes gear. The other thing which can be a bit startling is the noise of the aircraft engines in reverse thrust once the wheels have touched down. Again, this is perfectly normal and is done to assist the aircraft in stopping, very much as a car driver will change gear to help slow a car descending a steep hill.

Booking Your Seat

Okay, so I've got you up in the air with a drink in your hand and now I start talking about booking seats. The fact is that while it's easy for retired business people, who spent half their working lives in aircraft, to fly in retirement it's not quite as simple for those who've never flown before and it's best for them to have a vague idea of what to expect before they decide where to fly.

Mind you, booking our own tickets is where flying—like train travelling—becomes a whole new ball game for those of us who have had our business journeys planned and paid for—especially paid for— and I for one had as much to learn on that score as people who had never flown at all.

Making Friends with your Travel Agent
If you find a particularly helpful travel agent it's a good idea to give them a long-term view of your requirements. After trying them out for a couple of times you should call in at a quiet time and explain that you want to visit certain places and could be ready with just one week's, or even two or three day's, notice if a suitable bargain comes up. Stress the bargain aspect and that you are retired.

Molly's aunt snapped up a bargain fortnight in Greece when a travel agent friend rang her to say there was a last minute flight cancellation. She had less than a day's notice but cheerfully spent the afternoon buying sun tan lotion and a few other essentials, ironed and packed in the evening and was off next morning to somewhere she had never expected to visit.

Your agent can advise you about insurance, too, and can steer you away from tours of which there have been bad reports. Once you have established good relations with your travel agent you will find them invaluable for all sorts of travel, not just for package holidays by air.

If you haven't flown much before, or have done most of your flying at company expense, then calling on your travel agent could be the best move to make as soon as you start to think about flying in retirement. Agents make their money from commissions paid by tour operators, airlines and so on, which means that their own services to the traveller are absolutely free and although they are in the business to make money they have everything to gain by earning a reputation for giving good and impartial advice. Of course, much the same could be said about doctors and solicitors but that doesn't mean there are no quacks or crooked lawyers so it does pay to choose one's travel agent with care. There are a few basic rules—talk to friends, visit more than one agent if possible, avoid as a general rule agencies with patently sleazy disorganised offices and make absolutely sure—this is really important—that the agent you choose is a member of ABTA (Association of British Travel Agents). This membership ensures that, in the unlikely event of the agent doing a bunk or going out of business, you stand a good chance of getting back some or all of any cash you've paid out.

Naturally you can feel fairly certain that you'll be in good hands with one of the larger companies but you may feel, too, that you can expect more personal service from a smaller firm. Our friend, Paul Emery, who owns a travel agency and specialises in air travel, thinks that agents like himself can give retired people a lot of help. 'It's an important part of the travel agent's job to sift through the hundreds of brochures with which we are bombarded and to identify the best deal for older people who are a very important and growing section of our clientele. Of course we are not out to spoil the fun of looking through brochures when planning a trip—most people enjoy doing that themselves—but we can cut them down to half a dozen or so and, more important, we can go through the, often literally, small print.'

Who Flies Where

With package tours to the Mediterranean starting at under £100 you don't have to be all that wealthy to do at least some flying in retirement and, as Paul points out, 'You're talking about two hours from the English winter to the sunshine of Majorca. Chartered flights are always going to be cheaper than scheduled arrangements and often offer an additional advantage to older people of travel from their regional airport. There are package deals offering everything from a few days in the sun to most of the winter away for as little as £1.99 a day and retired people can pick up the best bargains because they are able to travel in the slack season—normally before and after Christmas.'

For people making their first flight in retirement a package deal could be the answer, after which there's a choice of remaining with the same sort of package, perhaps picking a different and more adventurous one or becoming more independent.

An intermediate step between package tours and complete independence is the 'seat-only' arrangement booked through a package operator. This could be useful, for example, if you have friends or relations who are able to offer you accommodation or if you have found some suitable cheap accommodation for yourself. It works in very much the same way as in the case of buses and coaches described earlier. However, some package tours, especially off season, are so cheap that if you took just the flight and forgot about food and accommodation it could still work out cheaper than any other way of flying there. If you do decide to do this you are obliged to tell your travel rep, which is not only good manners but stops people calling the police to report you missing.

On the whole, though, travel agents would rather book older people on package tours—unless they have their own villa or apartment or are definitely visiting friends—rather than seat-only, because when you are not with a group it's easy to forget things (like who is going to pick you up at the airport) and you yourself might be overlooked if there has to be a change in arrangements. And, while retired people do have time to do their own research, careless bargain hunters who decide to go it alone could find themselves taking a cheap 'sunshine' trip to Mombasa in April—the middle of the rainy season.

On most British and European routes it is simply not worth the hassle involved—especially for older people who haven't done a lot of flying—to try for any savings other than travelling by package tours, seat-only or by flying at off-peak periods when scheduled fares and airport charges may be cheaper. Even in Europe, however, retired people are usually able to book well in advance and to pick their times, which means they can take advantage of bargains that happen to be on offer. I found out about this the hard way when I had to fly to Nice on business without warning and discovered that the opulent looking chap in the next seat was flying with his wife for an inclusive stay at a first-class hotel for the same price I had paid for my ticket alone—a fact which very nearly spoiled the taste of my free champagne!

Long-Hauls and Bucket Shops

With so many bargains to be picked up legitimately it's hardly worth taking the slightest risk when booking short haul flights, but if you are travelling on long-haul flights, say to America or Australia or the Far East, the amount of money involved could make it worthwhile to look at the so called 'bucket shop' option.

Bucket shops are unlicensed travel shops which sell discounted tickets—bought in quantity from the airlines—to individual customers and they exist because the airlines that are members of the International Air Transport Association (IATA) have a couple of hundred million or so empty seats every year that they can't sell at the fixed prices they have agreed.

Technically, bucket shop proprietors are acting illegally and, though you are not breaking the law by buying discounted tickets in this way, it does reduce your chances of legal protection if anything goes wrong, although—as we shall see—retired people are better placed than most to minimise the risks.

Retired people are also well placed when it comes to finding a reliable bucket shop (which is not always easy as they are not entered under B in the Yellow Pages). Word of mouth is one good way of finding out and if you have friends who travel, say, to see children in Australia or a brother in Canada, on a regular basis they may well be able to help.

Some airlines, especially those operating in the Far East, will cheerfully give you the name of their 'consolidator' or buyer of discount tickets, provided you don't use the banned words 'bucket shop'. Older people who can manage to look ingenuous could get away with asking—after enquiries about the fare—'Oh dear! Isn't there somewhere I could get it a bit cheaper?'

Many smaller travel agents can supply discounted tickets, although they sometimes advise against them for older travellers on the grounds that they don't offer complete peace of mind, and one major company is trying to open its own discount section. Discount travel bargains are also on offer in 'quality' newspapers and some of the advertisers are in fact bucket shops. These adverts are well worth following. (If you can't afford to buy all the newspapers, check them in your local library reading room). Best newspapers are the *Times*, *Guardian*, *Daily Telegraph*, *Observer*, *Sunday Times* and *The Mail on Sunday*.

Small travel shops in or close to immigrant areas of large towns and cities, especially those with 'Travel Bargains' plastered over their windows, are often in the discount business. Their main trade lies in trips 'home' (which explains why many Asians use long-distance aircraft like other people use buses), but this doesn't mean they won't be happy to help anyone else as well.

Risks

Most bucket shop customers are well satisfied with their bargains—otherwise the shops would cease to exist—and the risk of being stranded or finding out that your flight doesn't exist is minimal. There is a very slight risk that your friendly bucket shop proprietor will go bust or decamp with the cash but this too can be minimised by those who take a few sensible precautions.

As far as I'm concerned the real risk in buying discounted tickets is of finding myself on a plane operated by a less than satisfactory carrier or discovering too late that the ticket has unacceptable restrictions—but these risks too can be avoided or minimised by checking in advance.

. . . and How to Avoid Them

First make sure that your bargain really is a bargain. Once you've found your 'discount agency' check the fares you are offered against those from the High Street travel agents with ABTA membership. Obviously, if there is only a little difference for precisely the same journey and airline it's not worth bothering with a bucket shop.

100

Try in the first instance to find bucket shops that are members of ABTA—in which case you get the best of both worlds—but this may be difficult as such shops are rare. Always check the airline on which the bucket shop proposes to book you. Avoid if possible Middle Eastern and African airlines and try for Australasian, North American or European. Don't pay more than a deposit—10 per cent is usual—until you've got your ticket in your hand and make sure that you can change your reservation or cancel your ticket once you have paid for it.

Pay for your ticket with Access or Visa credit cards, which will still give you protection under the Consumer Credit Act, but don't forget to top up your credit card before flying because it can be tremendously useful while you're away for paying hotel bills, buying presents and as a source of ready cash. If the bucket shop demands full payment up front, refuses credit cards or seems unwilling to provide the information you ask for, your best plan could be, as we used to say in the trade, to 'make an excuse and leave'.

Insurance

Although we talk about insurance in another chapter, it's worth emphasising that paying by credit card for your ticket might actually save you money—provided you pay off the amount quickly—because free insurance is often included if you pay that way. Of course, it pays to check that you are fully covered—medical expenses, particularly in America, are incredibly high even for minor things—but before you start paying out a high insurance premium find out from your own insurance company if you are partly covered under your household policy and how little they will accept to make up your full insurance cover. You may find that either credit card insurance or your own insurance company are cheaper than insuring through a travel firm but do make sure you are absolutely covered and take time out to check this thoroughly.

Open Sky

The price controls set by IATA have been easing and there is plenty of pressure in Britain and elsewhere to bring in an Open Sky policy. This calls for a fare structure largely influenced by market forces. However, in America, where many controls have recently been done away with, the results have not been totally happy. Some relaxation would have been good news for travellers with time to shop around but while competition is one thing, cut-throat competition is quite another and a completely Open Sky policy could lead to an unacceptable lowering of standards.

Meanwhile the totally legal fare offers already available include APEX (Advanced Purchase Excursion) and SUPER APEX for very long hauls to Australia and the Far East, PEX/SUPER PEX for short hauls, EXCURSION FARES for round trips on stipulated days and SPOUSE FARES where one spouse pays full fare and the other about half, usually with some restrictions like a requirement that husband and wife travel together. There are also ITX fares (which include accommodation) and STANDBY FARES.

Standby Fares

Standby fares can be useful savers for older people who are not in any hurry as they are valid only just before check-in time and provided that all the seats have not been booked in advance and taken. You can usually buy the actual standby tickets in advance or up to the last minute before the final check-in time but either way you are not guaranteed a seat on the aircraft or even a flight that day; and you also have to take the same sort of pot luck if you book a return standby. However, good reconnaissance can reduce the risk and there is something very satisfying about walking on to the same long-haul aircraft with a standby ticket as those who have paid full whack.

Standby is not the sort of thing I would think of unless I were a seasoned traveller, fit and healthy and actively enjoyed airports. Solo travellers often seem happy to book standby fares but if you are the sort of person whose blood pressure rises if your train or bus is ten minutes late a standby is not for you.

Air Passes

Some airlines sell Air Passes which allow unlimited air travel within a specific country—an obvious bargain for retired air travellers who can plan well in advance and thus make the most of them. Fly to America for example and you have a choice of airlines offering concessions on their domestic networks. Try to make sure, however, that the Air Pass is valid long enough for you to space out your flights as even bargain air travel can be tiring.

Whichever way you decide to fly, every airport—whether it's Luton or Las Vegas—is a gateway to excitement and every aircraft—whether it's a package charter or Concorde—is a magic carpet, taking you on what could be the trip of a lifetime.

Air Travellers Check List

(1)   Memorise your flight number *and* write it on a postcard
(2)   If being met on return—give them details of return flight number, date of return, arrival time, airline and tour company (if applicable) on a postcard
(3)   Keep luggage to a minimum but check if you need a warm jacket for mountain excursions and so on. Take a lightweight mac and some comfortable old shoes

(4) Arrive early at the airport—check coach, train or car will get you there early
(5) Double check money, credit cards, passport and address of destination
(6) Don't put your home address on your luggage, remove old labels and put on name and new destination only. LOCK YOUR LUGGAGE
(7) DON'T put cash, passport or valuables in your suitcase
(8) Take details of insurance and medical cover with you
(9) Check that you have your essential medical supplies (including any daily tablets or heart pills) with you in a small bag as well as larger amounts in your suitcase. This latter should include one full day's supply for the journey plus one extra day's supply in case of delay
(10) If you are travelling with a partner, make sure they know of any existing medical condition or medication. If travelling solo put these details on a postcard in your bag or pocket
(11) Make your final check calmly—leave key and addresses with neighbours or a relative. Don't leave your door open in a last minute mad rush
(12) Check that you have the correct number of pieces of luggage—three should be an absolute maximum, that is: suitcase, shoulder flight bag and handbag.
After that—relax.

Useful Addresses

Association of British Travel Agents, 55 Newman Street, London. Telephone (01) 637 2444. The people to complain to if you are not satisfied
Extrasure Insurance Services Limited, Lloyd's Avenue, London EC3N 3AX. Telephone (01) 488 9341. Recommended by ABTA

Further Reading

Exchange and Mart. A weekly newspaper, with a section on travel and travel bargains
Hogg Robinson Around the World Fares Planner, Hogg Robinson, London
Holiday Which?, Consumers' Association, London
The Complete Sky Traveller, David Beaty, Methuen, London. The good and bad of flying. How to cope, which seats to choose and so on. Details of the main British airports and how to get to them, including maps
The Round the World Air Guide, Katie Wood and George McDonald, Fontana. A comprehensive guide for travellers making a round-the-world trip, either on one ticket or several long-hauls. Ticket-buying, route planning advice and in-depth city reports, etc.
Time Out. London news and entertainment magazine which has the latest on travel bargains

10

Cut the Load — Cut the Worry

As the title of this chapter indicates, if you reduce what you have to carry then you have less to worry about. This applies not only to your physical load — luggage, etc. — but also to your mental load — worries about insurance, health and so on. Let us start where all journeys begin — packing our bags.

Packing

The best advice about packing that I've come across is to pack all the things you think you are going to need into suitcases and put all the money you think you'll need into your wallet; you then cut down the amount of gear by half and double the amount of money.

Of course it isn't always practicable to do exactly this — especially if money is tight — but the principle is sound and it's certainly a great deal easier for most older people to carry money or, preferably, traveller's cheques than to haul huge quantities of luggage about. This is especially true when things like toothpaste, shampoo, sun hats and so on can generally be purchased for about the same price abroad as they can be at home.

As a journalist I always used to keep a small bag packed with the absolute minimum for a foreign trip of a few days and if I had to stay away longer I would take the opportunity to stock up on new shirts and things. Now I am no longer working full-time, however, I find it pays to take more with me but at least I now have the time to make careful lists — which is helpful because these days I usually have a good idea of where exactly I'm going.

This wasn't always the case and one of my finest packing stories concerns the time when Molly and I were just setting off by car for my sister's wedding in Yorkshire with our clothes packed in two large suitcases. As we were leaving the house the 'phone rang and it was my

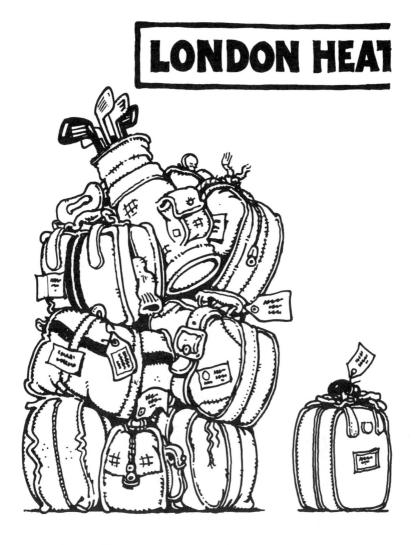

news editor telling me to drive to Grimsby immediately to board a ship for Iceland. I did manage to buy some fishing jerseys before sailing but had forgotten that Molly had split our clothes between the two cases and, as a result, I became one of the few chaps ever to sail to the Arctic with a large picture hat and a set of ladies underwear in a delicate shade of powder blue.

By contrast, retired people have the time to plan what they need to take with them and the best way to go about this is to make lists. Of course you also have time to pack well in advance but you have no need to overdo it as Molly's mother did when she invited us to join her for the last month of her winter stay in a Spanish apartment. She was found packing to come home on the day we arrived—a fact which put an immediate damper on our holiday!

Luggage

Before going into detail about what you want to pack it's a good idea to decide on the sort of luggage you are going to take. Of course this may well be influenced by what you have already but if your luggage is heavy and old fashioned—however good—it could be worthwhile buying new. Consider too the possibility of borrowing from a relative or friend, especially if you both only travel once or twice a year. On the other hand you will have to take responsibility for the luggage being returned in good condition and this could be a bit worrying— even if you are careful you can't guarantee that all the baggage handlers will be.

If you decide to get an orthodox suitcase, whether stiff or semi-stiff, the ones with built-in wheels are an absolute boon for older travellers but check that they have either an extending handle for pushing or a 'dog's chain' strap for pulling so that you don't have to stoop.

The next best thing is the wheel arrangement which can be hooked or strapped onto the case—although some of these need a little practise to fix on in a hurry—but either way, in these porterless days, if you have the slightest trouble carrying cases you need wheels.

You will find that when travelling in retirement you will often be helped by younger and fitter travellers. They are usually quite willing to help older people with luggage—provided they don't feel they are being exploited. Don't, for instance, assume because they are sitting next to you they will automatically fetch and carry for you on a long journey—unless of course they volunteer. If they are helpful the offer of a drink might be appreciated, but a grateful smile is usually quite sufficient.

If you know that you are not going to be able to manage on your own it's best to try to work out in advance how to deal with this. Obviously going solo with lots of changes is not for you but if you are travelling by rail, for instance, and let people know in advance, arrangements can often be made to help you. Coach tours where you are collected and delivered back home are excellent but check in advance that you are not expected to haul your own luggage about at stops *en route.* You have the time to sort out problems like this well beforehand and don't hesitate to write to tour companies with queries of this nature before you book.

However, arrangements can break down so it's not a bad idea to play the Worst Possible Scenario game and imagine yourself forced to deal with your own luggage — perhaps even having to get it up a flight of stairs all by yourself. It's not a particularly pleasing prospect but it isn't half a help when you are trying to decide whether or not you should pack that heavy pair of boots or your framed photos of the cat! So keep things light.

Personalising

Once you have decided on a suitcase one of the first things to do — unless it's already green with purple dots — is to customise or personalise it, and if you've ever watched the dance of the luggage carousel as people agonise over lookalikes you'll realise why. Paint flowers on your case, put go-faster stripes on it with coloured tape, stick on huge coloured initials, as Molly's mother did, or merely wrap a brightly coloured scarf tightly around the handle — just as long as you make it instantly identifiable as yours when it's brought out of the baggage compartment or the boot of a coach.

As well as a case it's a good idea to carry a reasonably sized item of hand luggage — preferably a shoulder bag — which you can take with you on coach, train, plane or boat, carrying the things you'll need *en route*. This too should be personalised.

Women travellers will probably also want a handbag for passport, money, travellers cheques, emergency medicaments, make up and so on. This makes the third item of luggage which is the ABSOLUTE MAXIMUM you should take; it's seldom possible to keep track of more than three pieces these days. The handbag should have a very secure fastening — Molly likes one which has several zipped compartments and a flap over the top which clicks fastened. It has both a shoulder strap and a wrist strap and is very lightweight. It's more difficult finding things in a bag with only one compartment, especially if you are feeling a bit flustered and think you've lost your glasses or your wallet. Incidentally, if you do wear glasses, it's a good idea to invest in one of those neck chains to hold them, otherwise you could lose a pair every time you travel.

Men travellers could find a jacket with lots of pockets is a good investment. It's best to make sure that the pockets are big enough to take, say, your passport and that some at least of the inside pockets are zipped for holding all the important extras like money and so on. A small briefcase is another choice, just as long as you make a point of ALWAYS keeping it with you.

What to Take

Before beginning to pack at all you should try to make certain that you know roughly what the weather is going to be like and to double check wherever possible. Travel agents often have 'average temperature' lists for different months at most resorts and you can generally work out approximately what your weather should be like. Of course there are times when these general figures are hopelessly wrong—it once rained every day of our holiday in southern Spain—but with a little judicious planning you can cater for most weather.

It's usually better to be too warm—you can always take your woolly off—than too cold and it's always best to take a light mac of some sort—I've landed in places like the Sunshine State in the pouring rain before now when the forecast said, 'Blue skies and eighty degrees'!

I usually travel in a heavy double cotton jacket with loads of big velcroed pockets and a couple of zipped ones; it's loose enough to be comfortable, the cotton is cooler than nylon but it fastens up to the neck if the weather is chilly. At the same time my shoulder bag—my current one is courtesy of Air France—holds an anorak, a pullover and anything else I might need on the journey. Naturally, being a bit of a cissy when it comes to the cold, if I know it's going to be really chilly—and travelling in winter even if you're on the way to sunshine can be very cold indeed—I take my big fur-lined jacket. After all, catching a chill on the journey is the best way to ruin your holiday.

I like to carry an emergency kit of essentials in my shoulder bag-hand luggage in case I get separated from my main luggage—which can happen. People's ideas about what is essential vary enormously but I always have a paperback book with me because I don't mind a delay if I have something to read and I make sure I have some boiled sweets, especially if I am flying, because not all airlines give you barley sugars and sucking sweets can prevent painful ear popping. Whenever Molly travels on her own, or when we go together anywhere, she takes food and drink in her shoulder bag. It can vary from a small snack to a full scale picnic and although I sometimes grumble and say we'll always be able to get something *en route* I have to admit that we're usually glad of her forethought. A hold up or breakdown while travelling in car, coach or train is made much more bearable if you can munch a sandwich and drink a hot cup of tea.

Coals to Newcastle

Naturally you'll want a tube of toothpaste with you when you travel any distance but just because you are going away for a month or so you don't really need to take several large tubes as—unless you are going to Outer Mongolia—you will probably find the same brand in the local supermarket. Except for Russia, China and a few other places that you can check out with your travel agent long before you go, you'll find toiletries, sun lotions, films, beach mats and so on readily available in the local shops. Of course if you are going to some remote spot you'll have to plan accordingly but you don't need to assume that there isn't a decent shop outside the British Isles! Canvas shoes and sun hats are often much cheaper abroad than in Britain and sun hats in particular are the most awkward things to pack. You may need a small canvas one for the journey but leave buying a large shady one until you arrive at your destination. Just remember that in most countries nowadays a supermarket is a supermarket is a supermarket and all you have to do is to pick up what you need; you don't even have to speak a word of the language.

One thing you may want to take with you, however, is a couple of packets of tea or some of your favourite tea bags as the cup that cheers is often much more expensive than at home and the brand to which you are addicted may not be available.

Knowing that almost everything you need is available in most industrialised or semi-industrialised countries means that you don't have to panic if you have forgotten the odd item. Even if you don't know the name for it in the local language you will probably find it in the supermarket. Provided you get yourself, your passport, your tickets and your money to wherever you want to go everything else can usually be begged, borrowed or bought. And as long as you get yourself safely to your destination even the loss of passport, tickets and money is not the end of the world, especially as you have more time to fix things and replace them than you would have as a time-restricted fully employed traveller. If you do lose important items, don't panic. This is where emergency postcards with the 'phone number of your insurance company and the number of your policy could be useful. One in your pocket and one in your bag is a good safety measure.

Unless you are rich enough not to care it's an idea to think carefully about the value of what you take with you when travelling and to think twice or even three times about the advisability of taking expensive jewellery.

Insurance

Some basic insurance is absolutely essential when travelling; after that is taken care of it's very much a question of what you are taking with you. Check VERY CAREFULLY with your broker or insurance agent—you may find you are covered for a certain amount under your ordinary household policy. If you are travelling on a package tour your Travel Agent or Tour Operator will explain what insurance, if any, is included in the cost. Check if you are fully covered for insurance if you pay for your trip by credit card. Make sure that you are still covered if your journey is delayed by a couple of days, for example, due perhaps to a strike. Some insurance cover is for a specific number of days and it pays to make absolutely sure that you are still covered in case of delay. Of course it goes without saying that the time to find out is before you book and not when you are sitting at Athens airport waiting for the traffic controllers to settle their dispute!

However else we may economise Molly and I always find the money for insurance cover somehow. This explains why, although we are both a bit excitable by nature, we usually look fairly laid-back when *en route*. The perils of not taking out insurance were brought home to Molly and her parents when she was a student and was taken ill with appendicitis on the French Riveria. Bills for an operation, followed by an extended stay for convalescence, made the whole family very careful about taking out insurance in the future. This paid off many years later when her mother had to be flown back from holiday in France and at least didn't have to worry about medical or transport bills.

We think that travel insurance is value for money if only for the peace of mind it brings with it and, looked at in that light, it's not too expensive. However, as we've said before, do check if you already have some cover under your ordinary policy or included in your tour and then take advice on any further cover you need.

Insurance Costs

A typical insurance policy from a reputable company is reassuring from the start because they are gambling that nothing is going to happen to you so they offer most cash for the things least likely to happen. Many insurance companies offer standard policies covering medical expenses up to about £250,000 which means that unless you were very unlucky you could even afford to be slightly poorly in America! The usual policy also covers baggage, a small amount for personal effects, life and accident insurance and cancellation insurance and, as well as taking care of medical bills, there is generally provision for getting you back home—by air ambulance if need be—should you fall ill. Regarding personal effects they consider us a pretty careless lot but they still offer something, say, £250. This emphasises our point about not taking valuable jewellery but, if you feel you simply must take your tiara, most insurance companies will make special arrangements.

At the same time most insurance companies are pretty certain that you aren't going to go out of your way to cause trouble so the personal liability clause they offer may well cover up to £1 million. Actually this is a very reassuring bit of insurance cover because if you were to be the innocent cause of an accident—especially abroad where the authorities may not be totally on your side—the cash is available. It also covers a point I would once have regarded as not being all that important—providing money for the necessary arrangements to be made should you be unfortunate enough to die while on your travels. This does worry quite a lot of people as I found out when I went on a Young At Heart trip to Spain. I discovered that some people spending a long time there had recently visited an old-style mausoleum and were very concerned that they too might finish up as some part of a foreign wall. Firstly, of course, there was no way the tour company was going to allow this to happen and, secondly, the sort of insurance policy I've mentioned would allow about £1,000 for appropriate burial expenses abroad or transport back to Britain.

If you are booking through tour agents you will probably find that they have either an 'insurance included' section on your booking form—in which case you should check carefully exactly what is covered—or you will be able to purchase holiday insurance at special rates through them with a reputable insurance company.

Thomson's Young At Heart holidays can be covered very reason-ably by a special Norwich Union policy arranged by the tour com-pany. It's particularly aimed at the long-stay traveller and provides full insurance—even to emergency funds if your luggage should be delayed—from £15.35 for up to 9 nights to only £35 for long stays of 64 days and over. These rates apply to all the Young At Heart winter holidays in places ranging from the Algarve to Tunisia and are probably the most economical you would find.

When I was working for other people full-time I suppose I must have been over insured on most of my journeys but, as a belt and braces sort of person, I didn't worry too much about that. Nowadays I tend to check to see whether I'm insuring myself twice over for the same risk and for all retired people the aim should be to get the best possible coverage for the least possible outlay. You have the time to check just what you are entitled to as part of any package deal and if you don't think you have enough cover you can consult your insurance agent and build up from there.

Reciprocal Medical Arrangements

Of course as *bona fide* travellers in retirement we are going to make absolutely certain that we get any free or low cost medical treatment we may need to which we are entitled—after all, we have paid for it in Britain through our National Health contributions.

As a national of, and resident in, Britain and the European Com-munity you are entitled to emergency medical treatment either free or at reduced cost when visiting other Community countries. If you need treatment while you are abroad and want to claim under these rules you will need to produce a Certificate E111 together with Leaflet SA 30 *Medical Costs Abroad*. You can obtain both from the DHSS. They will usually tell you that you can obtain the forms from your local office but in practice they have often run out, so it's best to apply for the forms well in advance.

The Certificate E111 entitles you to treatment in Belgium, Denmark, France, West Germany, Gibraltar, Greece, Italy, Luxembourg, the Netherlands, Portugal and Spain while in the Irish Republic you don't have to bother with forms. Other countries which have agreements with Britain for free or reduced treatment in emergencies are: Australia, Bulgaria, the Channel Isles, Czechoslovakia, Finland, East Germany, Hong Kong, Iceland, Malta, New Zealand, Norway, Poland, Romania, Russia, Sweden and Yugoslavia. In these countries your passport is regarded as sufficient proof of entitlement.

Keep the Bills

Customs vary and in some places you may be required to pay the bill first and claim a refund afterwards so it's very important to make sure that you or someone with you asks for and keeps all bills and receipts for treatment. Of course you would also need these if you have to make a claim against your insurance policy.

Don't be a White Rabbit

Although it sounds a bit complicated, insurance policies are really designed to save worry over things like losing bits and pieces of luggage and getting ill while we're away from home.

Of course this doesn't mean that we no longer have to think about such things but it does mean that we've no need to get into a state about them. In fact, as travellers in retirement we have no real need to get into a state about anything.

I must confess that I used to be a White Rabbit Traveller—remember the harrassed White Rabbit in *Alice Through the Looking Glass* who hurried along mumbling, 'Oh my ears and whiskers! I'm late, I'm late . . .'—but a couple of trips to southern Ireland changed all that. At first I found the slow pace absolute hell and it took me a while to realise that I was the one out of step. The Irish didn't seem to worry unduly about things that couldn't be helped and they always had time for a drink and a chat.

It's a good plan to take things easy, not to worry about things being 'different' from at home or get upset when things go wrong as they are bound to do on occasions. One travel company among those who specialise in travel for older people actually breaks the mould by abandoning the lyrical approach to foreign parts favoured by their competitors; they go out of their way to stress that part and parcel of going abroad is that things are certainly not going to be exactly as we like them at home. Often of course they will be better but, for example, if we go to places where it's very sunny we can expect the occasional water shortage, the food may not be what we are used to, things may not always work—and it may even rain. Enjoy the differences, they say, after all, that's part of what you are travelling for.

For reassurance that you are not alone, and that things could be a great deal worse, you could read *Great Holiday Disasters* which will at least make you chuckle.

Be a Boy Scout

Worrying is bad—being prepared on the other hand is good. Ask your travel agent about special health precautions—if any—for wherever you are going and if you have any special medical problem check with your doctor before leaving.

Long-Standing Conditions

If you have a particular medical condition—angina, diabetes and so on—and are taking medicines it is a good idea to have a note from your doctor describing your condition and your medication. You should also discuss with your doctor, especially if you are going away for several months, whether you should take sufficient tablets and so on for the entire period or whether you should obtain them abroad. Usually it's best to take them with you but don't forget to have a small supply of *everything* you need in your hand luggage. Molly's mother made up a set of small white drawstring bags for medical supplies when travelling. One with a red cross was for ordinary things like soluble aspirin, sting relief cream, elastoplasts, anti-diarrhoea tablets and so on; the second with a blue cross was for Harry's tablets and medicines which he had to take regularly for a heart condition, while a very small one with a blue cross held two small plastic bottles, each with a day's supply.

If you are disabled or very frail you need to make your requirements known well in advance, telling people exactly what help you need on the journey and when you get to your destination. Be absolutely honest about your condition and what you need, especially with regard to special diets, access ramps and so on otherwise your trip could be disappointing and frustrating. If you have a disability and want to travel—planning is all.

The Disabled Traveller

There is a tremendous amount of information about special facilities available for disabled travellers—it's just a question of knowing where to get hold of it. So, we mention here two publications which we think are virtually essential.

The AA Travellers' Guide For The Disabled is published by the AA and is free to members, although non-members can obtain it from bookshops. It is a complete guide on where to go and where to stay in Britain, plus a lot of useful information on travel abroad. *The Disabled Traveller's International Phrase Book* from the Disability Press, has a vocabulary you might not find in most phrase books.

We can't stress enough, however, that careful and detailed planning is the key to an enjoyable holiday if you are disabled. It pays to check that 'wheelchair access' doesn't just mean to your room on the ground floor if the bar or entertainments room is on the floor above—in other words, take the time to write or telephone to make sure that all the basic things you require are available.

Care Home Holidays

Even people who are in need of special care can enjoy travel and a break from routine by taking advantage of a network of specialist care homes organised in consultation with Help the Aged. These homes are for people who need the sort of nursing and medical attention provided either in the family home or in nursing homes—24-hour emergency facilities, night staff and chambermaids who are experienced care attendants. The organisation offers both Rest Homes—where you can get the sort of care you'd expect to receive from a caring relative in a family home—and Nursing Homes which offer full nursing care.

Costs at the Rest Home type of accommodation are generally based on a 7-day week with not a few former stately homes on offer, even in the middle range, and even though classified as 'Rest Homes' many also offer a lot more in respect of nursing facilities than most 'caring relatives' could provide.

The Nursing Homes are also based on a 7-day stay and many offer extras such as house cars and so on. Transport, ranging from ambulances to a car to meet you at the station, can be arranged and a courier will make at least one call on you during your stay as well as coping with any queries. This option could be useful if you are not up to going off by yourself or away with the family. If your family have been nursing you for some time they too will probably appreciate a break as much as you appreciate travelling off to somewhere new.

Health En Route

After you've consulted your doctor about any existing medical condition and checked well in advance with your tour operator about any possible vaccinations required for far off places there are two conditions most likely to interfere with travel plans and travel enjoyment—diarrhoea and sunburn.

Both of these can be prevented to a large extent. To prevent diarrhoea it's very definitely a question of being careful about what you eat and drink—especially in hot countries—and of taking immediate action if you have any trouble. Take water-purifying tablets with you and a bottle of medicine. We've also found that mint tisanes in little teabags are a first-class way of settling the stomach after any attack. If none of these works get help immediately, preferably from an English-speaking doctor who will probably be used to this happening and should have a first-class remedy.

As to sunburn—I used to go round looking like Rudolf the Red Nosed Reindeer every summer until I started using a sun cream with the right filter factor and now I have no trouble at all, but perhaps that's also because I now treat the sun with a bit more respect than I used to and don't lie in it for hours. Touch wood, I haven't had a real medical emergency abroad since we got married, although we did once have to get the vet to Molly! (Thanks to some currency exchange problems, when living in France we were too poor to be able to pay a doctor. The local vet, who charged less, came out and treated Molly for her pleurisy.)

Fortunately few of us should need the doctor—or the vet—because travel in itself will help to keep us healthy by encouraging us to take more exercise, providing a beneficial change of climate and getting us away from the strains and tensions of our everyday lives.

Travel in retirement in other words could easily keep us fitter and help us live longer than might be the case if we remained at home. It certainly helps make life a great deal more enjoyable.

Basic Checklist

Suitcase
Wheels—personalised—name and destination only on label
Contents: shoes—clothes—towel—teabags

Hand Luggage
Lightweight—shoulder strap—lockable—personalised—name and destination only on label
Contents: toilet bag—tube of Easy Wash—face cleansers—mini

towel—pullover or cardigan—lightweight anorak—food for journey—two cup flask—paperback book—medical kit—main supply of
tablets—change of underwear—duplicate postcards with vital phone
numbers

Handbag or Briefcase or Jacket Pockets
Passport—tickets—travellers cheques—phrase book—tiny supply of
essential tablets—travel sickness pills—aspirin—boiled sweets—
glasses—sun glasses—needle and cotton—postcards with vital phone
numbers—small cotton sun hat

Useful Addresses

Association of British Insurers, Aldemary House, Queen Street, London
EC4N 1TT. Ask for the free holiday insurance brochure

Care Home Holidays Limited, Wern Manor, Porthmadog, Gwynedd, Wales.
Short stay holiday breaks for people who need special care. A wide range

DHSS Leaflet Unit, Stanmore, HA7 1AY. This is the best place to obtain
leaflets which your local DHSS may have run out of or are unable to supply
in time for your trip. You will need *Medical Costs Abroad* as it includes—
detachable from the leaflet—the application form for Certificate E111.
Also ask for *Protect Your Health Abroad*

Help the Aged, St James' Walk, London EC1R 0BE. Telephone (01) 253
0253

Holiday Care Service, 2 Old Bank Chambers, Station Road, Horley RH6
9HW. Useful free advice about holidays for the elderly and disabled

RADAR (The Royal Association for Disability & Rahabilitation), 25
Mortimer Street, London W1N 8AB. Publishes access guides and has a
holiday insurance package

Further Reading

AA Traveller's Guide for the Disabled, Automobile Association, Basingstoke. A
first-class comprehensive guide with masses of useful information

AA Traveller's Guide to Europe, Automobile Association, Basingstoke. Lots of
useful information

Choice. A magazine for the retired. Articles, helpful advice and information.
Obtainable from the publishers, Choice Magazine, Bedford Chambers, 19
Undine Street, London

Great Holiday Disasters, Perrott Phillips, Christopher Helm, London

Holiday Which?, Consumers' Association, Caxton Hill, Hertford

The Disabled Traveller's International Phrasebook, Disability Press, 60 Green-hayes Avenue, Banstead SM7 2JA. Invaluable for any disabled traveller. Information and phrase words not usually found in similar phrasebooks

Travel Which?, Consumers' Association, Caxton Hill, Hertford. Useful for tips and up-to-date information

11

Safety on the Move

Ever since people began to travel there have been villains around ready to capitalise on the fact that folk on the move were vulnerable, as they were forced to take money and valuables with them, which made them easy pickings for footpads and highwaymen.

Nowadays nothing has changed, except that more older people are travelling and you might think that they would make particularly tempting targets for the criminal. After all, we do tend to get weaker as we get older and therefore less able to offer resistance. In fact you would be wrong, as the people most likely to be victims of violent crime are young men between the ages of 16 and 20.

Security

When it comes to security, making things difficult for the criminal is the name of the game and not only do most older people have more sense than the majority of youngsters when it's a question of their own safety but they usually have more time to think about security measures.

Retired travellers—if they did much travelling before leaving full-time work—have usually evolved their own security plans but now they have the time to reassess them, add to them where necessary and work out the sort of check lists we older people find increasingly useful.

Of course, it's mainly a matter of common sense but if everyone behaved sensibly half the policemen in the world could join the ranks of the retired. As it is Crime Prevention is one of the most flourishing branches of police forces, while private security is a growth industry — which at least means that we can let the travelling retired millionaires look after their own security problems.

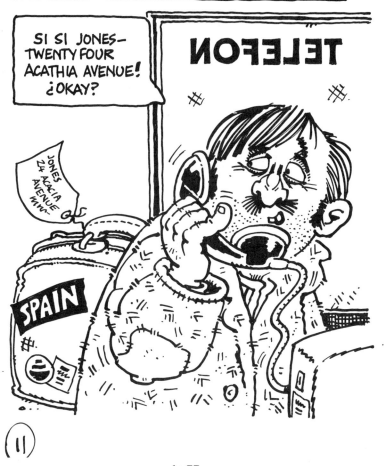

At Home

Remember—security begins at home. If you are travelling in retirement it will often mean that you are away from home well outside the usual holiday times but, although this is interesting local gossip, don't tell everyone in the pub that you are going away and for how long.

Tell your neighbours and friends of course—they'll find out anyway and will act as an unofficial neighbourhood watch on your behalf.

119

Don't forget to tell your nearest and dearest if you intend being away for any length of time as they might otherwise begin to worry when they do not receive a reply to letters and 'phone calls; and do make sure that a trusted neighbour has your forwarding address, if there is one, or some way of reaching you if you are touring. One way of keeping in touch is to arrange to make a regular check call to someone, even if it's only once a month, which won't cost too much from most countries with direct dialling—as long as you resist the temptation to chat.

Do make sure your insurance is in order and try to store any valuables in a place of safety or, if this is impossible, let the police know that you are leaving your house unattended—not a bad idea in any case if you are going to be away for a long time.

We always left a key with one of our neighbours who acted as unofficial house minder while we were away for months, and even years, at a time but we are perhaps a little less selfish these days and find it fairer to make an arrangement with friends who intend going away at different times to watch each others houses.

Take time for a correspondence session and, if you are going away for a couple of months or so, you might think about leaving the telephone instrument with a neighbour—if you have one of the modern plug-in versions—as it's hardly likely that even the most farsighted miscreant would arrive complete with his own 'phone, prepared to contact his auntie in Australia.

Make a list of the *obvious* things to do before leaving the house:

Cancel milk
Cancel papers
Close windows and check catches
Bolt back and side doors if any
Switch water off at the main tap—if you don't know where it is or
    can't shift it then ask a neighbour for help but if the tap is outside
    make sure you leave a torch in some convenient place if you
    arrive back in the middle of the night and are desperate for a cup
    of tea
Make sure all the lights and electrical appliances are switched off
    and all gas fires and pilot lights are turned off completely

If you have a Rubens—or for that matter a Jackson Pollack—in your hall and don't want to leave them in the bank or somewhere safe it could be worthwhile consulting your local crime prevention officer or a reputable security firm. One of the cheapest security 'gimmicks' is a time-switch which will turn on your lights and radio every so often but you can also install many different types of alarm if you feel the need. On the whole though it might be better to move valuables to a safe place.

Double check everything before leaving home and allow time for this, even checking off a list; the old joke about wondering whether you left the gas on when you're flying at 20,000 feet is still fairly amusing but not if it happens to you.

Cash and Credit Cards

You will have to carry some cash with you and as you are likely to be among milling crowds, some of whom may have designs on your belongings, you should refrain from tempting fate by waving all your money around in a huge wad. Even at low season, when you will probably be doing most of your travelling, boats, airports, trains and supermarkets are still crowded.

I usually decide on the amount of British currency I'm going to need for, say, the journey to the airport and all requirements until I get to my destination. I then add about half as much again for extra drinks, minor delays and so on, putting the sum in question into two easily getatable pockets, one of which buttons down. On the opposite side of my jacket in a similar pocket I put the amount of foreign currency I'm going to need to get to my hotel—which could in fact be very little—and then add half as much again. Then in an inside zipped pocket I put the major part of my foreign currency, together with my travellers cheques and in a separate one—preferably zipped or buttoned—I keep my cheque card and credit card.

Of course if you are touring and maybe passing through two or three countries you'll want to keep the currencies separate and the plastic change envelopes from your bank are quite useful for this, provided you put different coloured slips of paper on each one marked with French, Italian, Spanish and so on. Large freezer labels in different colours will stick well to the plastic. The actual arrangement of course is a matter of personal choice but the main thing is not to carry everything of value in one pocket or bag and to avoid flashing large sums by keeping relatively small amounts of 'pocket money' conveniently close to hand.

Handbags, especially those with lots of compartments, are very useful and it's tempting to put absolutely everything in one—many men now carry a masculine version with money, passport, tickets, credit cards, the lot, all nice and handy. The trouble is that they are also handy for bag snatchers and even though they often come with a wide wrist strap—which is safer than a shoulder strap—it still doesn't seem a good idea to keep everything in one place.

Money belts are not a bad idea for papers and money you are not going to need *en route* but do make sure they definitely won't be needed until you arrive—if only to avoid a last minute dash to the loo or an embarrassing striptease.

Hal Newell has what he calls an 'Aussie pouch' firmly achored to his

121

belt with a metal key arrangement and carries most of his money and important papers in it. It also has a zip fastener and a snap down flap which in some parts of the world—Cairo for instance—is double security against pickpockets. Hal also claims that the holster-like arrangement saved not only his money but perhaps his life when he was last in America and found himself threatened by three obvious hard cases while walking through Harlem. He pushed back his jacket to reveal the leather pouch and backed off at speed while his potential assailants were still wondering how quickly he could draw and fire! Mind you, the fact that Hal looks and talks like an older version of Crocodile Dundee might have had something to do with it and even he realises that he was fortunate to get away unscathed.

Luggage
Apart from not telling all and sundry that you are going away—as we mentioned earlier—you should also refrain from letting everyone at airports and coach stations know your home address and the fact that your house may be empty. They can easily deduce this if you cover your luggage with labels clearly marked with your name and home address. Most travel experts recommend that you write your name and address on a postcard in block capitals and put it inside your suitcase, together with your destination when you are just setting off. That way even if your luggage ends up in Delhi while you are in Paris you stand a chance of getting it back.

Identifying your luggage among a mass of similar bags and cases can sometimes be a bit of a problem; as we've mentioned before Molly's mother used to put her own personal logo on all her baggage—a bold monogram of her initials in different coloured scotch tape. As she admitted, it looked a bit flashy but she could pick out her own cases even without her glasses. It also helps in identification if someone should mislay your stuff.

Hotels
If there's one thing worse than having to worry about security while travelling, its having to think about it when you arrive at your destination, whether it's a hotel, a guest house, an apartment or a camping site. Worst of all is wondering what you should take while you explore the town or go to the beach, but at least retired people have the time to give security a bit of thought without having to cope with impatient kids who want to get into the water before you've drawn breath.

Personal Safety

As soon as you arrive, check out your escape route in case of fire. Of course this applies to people of all ages but it's particularly important for older people who may not be as agile as youngsters. Make sure that the fire doors will open from the inside and kick up a great fuss if they don't. Fix in your mind whether the escape route is left or right of your room and how many doors away. Check also whether it's possible to get out of your window in an emergency. By that I mean whether it opens and if there is a balcony outside.

For older people it's a good idea to insist on being no higher than the fourth floor of a building. For one thing, if the lifts are out of order for any reason, you don't want to be huffing and puffing up to the top floor—leave that to younger people—and, for another, fire brigade ladders don't reach higher than the fourth floor. Make your requirements known very firmly—after all it's not high season and you don't have to be put off because the hotel is double booked or people are sleeping on the beaches because there isn't a room to be had.

Valuables

The first rule of course is to take as few valuables as possible whenever you travel and the second is to know exactly what you have with you. This may sound ridiculous but if you are used to wearing different rings and earrings and have two or three watches it could be difficult to remember whether you have really lost them or if you left them at home. This is where a list comes in useful but not, obviously, one which details 'gold watch' or 'sapphire ring'; some sort of personal code, even as simple as 3R, 4E—indicating that you have taken 3 rings and 4 sets of earrings—would do.

Many hotels and guest houses have security safes and if you are going out for the day it's as well to leave valuables in them. Some hotels have personal safes in guests' rooms and these are well worth using—even the ones where you have to put in the equivalent of a couple of pounds in the slot for the key. Of course in this case you are advertising just where your valuables are but most hotel thefts are opportunistic and it would take a fairly determined thief to crack even the flimsiest safe. Not only that but you would know immediately that you had been robbed—and not merely mislaid things—and could notify the hotel manager, your travel agent's rep, if there is one, the local police, your bank, your insurance company and your credit card company.

Of course, as a careful traveller, you will have all the relevant information immediately available on cards which you will not—as we once did—have carefully locked away in the safe! In fact it's just as well to have at least two copies of emergency numbers and information spread about your belongings; one maybe in your pocket or bag and another, say, at the bottom of the dirty laundry bag.

Your list should include addresses and phone numbers for:

Insurance Company
Let them know straight away either by 'phone or letter, depending on the value of what has been taken and make sure they know the matter has been reported to the local police.

Local Police
Someone else will almost certainly call them but include it just in case.

Bank
Always try to remember not to keep your cheque card and cheque book together, but if they both get stolen or are lost it's a good idea to telephone the bank. Then follow this up immediately with a confirming letter.

Credit Card Companies
Telephone as soon as possible giving the numbers of your card—keep this information on your list next to their 'phone numbers. If the company, or your bank, has a local branch office it's a good idea to contact them first as with a bit of luck they might deal with everything for you, but they will need details of your cards. We take only one credit card when we go abroad, which makes us look like poor relations—especially in America—but it would save an awful lot of trouble if we were to be robbed.

Doctor
Keep your doctor's address and 'phone number on the same card, plus the local doctor's number if you are staying for any length of time.

It might all sound like a lot of trouble for nothing and of course you are almost certainly *not* going to be robbed, unless you count someone nicking your towel or sun tan oil from the beach or pool. Even if you are robbed you will probably find the hotel staff or local agent will put through calls for you, but with your information list you'll feel more secure and you'll be able to sort things out much more quickly and efficiently if it does happen. Incidentally, nothing persuades hotel staff and others to be helpful in times of emergency more than a rueful smile, quiet persistence—and a handful of local currency.

Caravan and Camping Security

This is a bit difficult and if you are staying in a tent there is really nowhere safe for your valuables. The best thing is to take as few as possible and keep them with you or ask the site owner to put them in his safe.

In a caravan you can make things difficult for would-be thieves by making sure your locks are efficient and using them even when you go out for a short while. Don't leave a window open—even a small one—and don't leave radios, jewellery or a handbag in a temptingly visible place. Molly's father, who was a useful handyman, soldered a lockable metal container to the base of their caravan inside one of the lift-up seats. The particular seat was then secured with a couple of screws. It's not something to do for things you need everyday but it is useful for insurance papers and travellers cheques and so on and gives a little added security.

No-go Areas

It's a sad fact of life that most big cities and larger towns have areas into which it's unwise for a stranger to venture. You wouldn't usually wander round such a district in your own country so if you're abroad—play it safe. If it looks a tough neighbourhood, treat it as such.

Of course there are parts of the world—like the Reeperbahn in Hamburg and Amsterdam's Outezijds Voorburgwal, and the much lamented Bougis Street in Singapore—where parts of the Red Light Districts have been turned into tourist attractions, but apart from places like these the best way to treat tough areas is to stay away from them.

When in a strange city at night, don't go out by yourself, keep to the well lighted streets, walk well away from the wall and in the middle of the pavement, where possible, and always walk as if you know exactly where you are going. Save sauntering for the daytime unless you are with an organised group.

I hate to say this but if you are really old and infirm you shouldn't walk the streets at night at all in most big cities—Singapore, unless it has changed recently, is a shining exception and some of the Eastern Bloc cities are regarded as generally crime free, but apart from these you need to be in a large group to be safe.

Cars and Taxis

Taxis are usually fine and for a reasonable tip the drivers will often be knowledgeable tourist guides, advising you against places where they think you ought not to go and suggesting others where you can enjoy yourself safely.

If you are in your own car or a hired car make sure you lock the doors—even when you are in the car—and close the windows fully at any sign of trouble. This is unlikely in most places but it's just as well to be prepared and to know what to do. When you leave the car, check the doors, windows and boot, not forgetting the sun roof, always take out the ignition key and, at night, park under a light if possible. Don't leave documents in the car and if you do have to leave anything of value it's best to lock it away in the boot. Try not to leave valuable gear on the roof rack but if you have to, say while you're having a meal *en route*, make sure that it's firmly tied down—a lockable chain stretched over the top could deter a casual opportunistic thief.

If it's your own car, the police and motoring organisations also recommend locking petrol caps and wheel nuts and for new cars they suggest etching the registration number on all the windows. For an older car which may have no steering lock it's worth using a steering clamp or fitting an immobiliser or an alarm.

Safety First, Second and Third

Think safety and security! Don't be put off because it sounds too depressing for words. The plain fact is that accidents do happen and there are some bad guys about who don't advertise the fact with striped jerseys and swag bags so you can avoid them. Even young people get mugged. My judo instructor had his jaw broken by muggers who took him by surprise and although in the end they were very sorry indeed that they had picked on him it didn't do much to lessen his pain.

He might not have been attacked at all if he had been playing *The Worst Possible Scenario* (WPS) game instead of thinking up fresh tortures to inflict on his students in the name of exercise.

The WPS game covers all situations where safety and security are matters for concern and is simply a question of imagining what is the worst thing that might happen in any given circumstance—and being prepared for it. The beauty of it is that, as you are invariably the hero or heroine of your own game, your responses are always geared to your own physical and mental capabilities. For example, you are about to set off on holiday: imagine the Worst Possible Scenario.

Worst Possible Scenario Number One
A burglar targets your house. Have you done enough to make your house secure? Have you asked the police for their leaflet, *Holiday Watch*, and for any details on their local Good Neighbour Scheme? Have you put your valuables somewhere safe—is a reliable neighbour or relative keeping an eye on the place. Go through your check lists and make certain.

Worst Possible Scenario Number Two
A burglar has broken into your home despite your precautions. Are you insured, are your valuables photographed and marked? Do the police or your neighbour have an address or telephone number where you can be reached? With one of those instant picture cameras—which are quite cheap—you could photograph your jewellery, silver, china, pictures and so on in an afternoon and missing items are much more likely to be returned if there is a photograph rather than a vague description. Don't leave the photographs lying around, however. It's best to put them in a sealed envelope and leave them at the bank while you're away.

Worst Possible Scenario Number Three
A coach crash while touring or travelling to the airport. Of course the odds are very much against it happening but if you play the WPS game you will know where the emergency doors are in relation to your seat.

Worst Possible Scenario Number Four
In a plane the WPS is obviously a crash but it's reassuring to remember that flying is much safer than crossing the road. Even so it's worthwhile being the only people on the plane who really listen to the stewardess's instructions on how to put on a lifejacket, how to use an oxygen mask and where the emergency doors are. Don't be afraid to ask her to repeat the instructions if you didn't quite catch them. Fine, so it's a million to one chance, but if you're travelling in retirement it pays to play safe.

Worst Possible Scenario Number Five
A hotel fire. In the hotel or guest house, play the WPS game right from the start. Tell the receptionist that you are superstitious about occupying a room above the fourth floor—unless of course you are on the top floor with access to the roof. If you have a slight heart condition it's best in any case to be near the ground floor in case of a failure in the electricity supply which, apart from anything else, will stop the lifts. Try to check out the fire exit and fire stairs as soon as you arrive anywhere and make sure that the fire escape hasn't been padlocked to prevent burglars getting in.

The WPS game can be described as constructive worrying and as such is warmly recommended by police and security experts. The point is that if you have worked out what you are going to do if the worst happens it almost certainly won't.

Worst Possible Scenario Number Six
Mugging. Although the odds are against it, you might consider the WPS factor in terms of mugging in a strange city. Here the main thing

is to keep cool in the first instance and if there's no one around to help you and the choice is 'your money or your life'—*always* give them the money. Okay, so it hurts to part with your pension money, all your tour spending money or your life savings—which you shouldn't have had with you in the first place—but you are more important than your money. 'Having a go' is risky at any age but when you are older it can be suicidal.

Of course if it's your life rather than your property which is in danger then you have to make another quick decision. Scream and shout like mad, for a start—wake up the whole neighbourhood if you can and if you're lucky your assailant may break and run. If shouting doesn't work then try breaking glass—any glass—house window, shop window; there are few sounds more difficult to ignore than the noise of plate glass shattering and a walking stick, if you use one, can be very useful for this.

Most crime is committed by opportunist criminals who don't want to work hard and don't really want a lot of trouble and it's useful to remember that it's always better to lose your possessions than your life and better to walk away than stand your ground and finish up lying on it, but if you don't have a choice then don't be squeamish—be prepared to hit out very hard—maybe a jab on the kneecaps or hard under the nose—anything to give you time to get away or get help. Shouting, 'Fire' is always useful and making for a well lit cafe or pub.

Best of all defences is to avoid, if possible, situations where you are vulnerable and on your own.

Safety in Numbers

There's definitely safety in numbers and this applies particularly to older people. Whether you are caravanning, cycling, touring by coach, train or plane it's best to keep within reach of other people and if you are definitely a 'solo' traveller then take a few sensible precautions and don't decide to do your exploring just as it's getting dark.

With a bit of luck you won't have to deal with any of the Worst Possible Scenarios in reality but a little bit of forethought could make you more confident, less likely to panic in an emergency and able to take control of the situation to the full extent of your capabilities both physical and mental.

12

You Don't Have to Speak
the Language

'You don't have to speak the language . . .' as the old song has it, and it's perfectly true that if you wish to express a romantic interest in someone it can usually be managed without words. However, if you want to ask the way to the nearest public toilet in a country where you don't speak a word of the language you could be in for a few embarrassing moments. Mind you, there are people to whom this doesn't apply and Molly's father was one of them, largely I suspect because he was a complete extrovert who didn't know the meaning of the word embarrassment and whose sole aim was simply to get his message across.

Harry's great advantage—apart from his supreme unconcern for what other people might think of him—was his decidedly un-English appearance, a legacy of an Italian grandmother which, for some reason, put foreigners at their ease and smoothed the path for his mime performance. Foreigners, especially children, were immediately aware that he was enjoying himself hugely and within minutes of starting a 'conversation' he was surrounded by smiling locals, convulsed by his efforts to order eggs by drawing ovals in the dust with a stick and flapping his arms, while making clucking noises. They laughed . . . but he always got his eggs.

Like many people of his generation Harry missed out on formal language tuition but he realised instinctively that things like love, laughter and hunger are universal and that when it's a question of expressing basic needs you can't afford to be shy. Unfortunately, most of us who have reached retirement age now realise that even if we attended classes in French or German or Spanish at school we were often so badly taught that we not only forgot most of it but were put off languages completely. This, combined with the notion that 'English people are bad at languages' has often been enough to kill any ambition to communicate with foreigners stone dead. We older

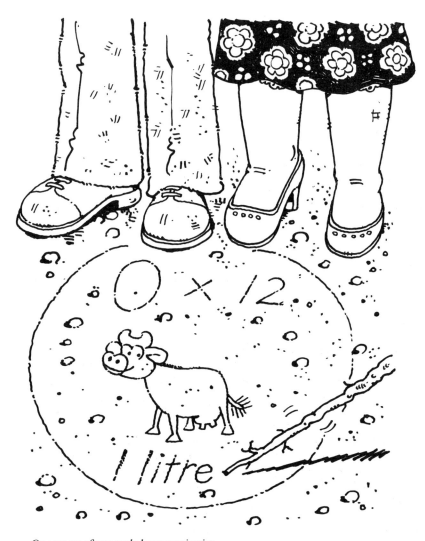

One means of non-verbal communication . . .

people are among the most disadvantaged in this respect but at least being retired enables us to redress the situation.

One thing older folk share with young children is that we needn't be shy. Worrying about what other people think is a barrier to communication and retired people should be old enough to know better! Another thing—we are probably better motivated than most of us were as schoolchildren. After all, the thought of being able to order a coffee or a beer in a foreign country is a more powerful incentive than trying to avoid the teacher's displeasure by mugging up irregular verbs.

Being British Helps

If English is your native tongue you are quids in when travelling to foreign parts—mainly because, as the world's most widely spoken language after Mandarin Chinese, English is understood by more than 400 million people. Few of them will understand you much better if you shout, however, so you will stand a better chance of being understood if you speak clearly. Of course, you should make sure you're not talking to an Oxbridge graduate before speaking as if to a backward child.

Having English as one's mother tongue has another advantage because if you are old enough to be retired you already have a considerable vocabulary in many foreign languages without even being aware of it. For one thing English is such a mixture of languages that many words are shared anyway; and, for another, English is so wide-spread that many languages have borrowed words from it, while within human memory British soldiers and administrators looted words from every country they occupied.

The Normans provided the English with hundreds of French words, although the fact that the English at that time were a subject race who looked after the animals while the Normans ate them is subtly indicated by the fact that English words for mutton, beef and pork reflect the French words for live animals. Older people, especially those who recall words like chota peg, Memsahib, ayah and bungalow—not to mention Army expressions like char, and san-fairy-ann—have a large foreign vocabulary and it's a comfort to come across old friends even in places like Romania where so much else seems alien.

Romania is a delightful example of the advantages to be gained by picking up a smattering of a few European languages because in its most simplistic form it seems a bit like dyslexic Esperanto. For example, a knife is a 'cutit', a lift is an 'ascensor', lunch is 'dejun' and meat is 'carne', while garage is 'garaj', a cigarette is a 'tigara' and shaving cream is 'crema de raz'. Of course there are some of what the French call *faux amis* (false friends) among the words that seem alike but not many people are going to be too worried if 'pantofi'—which they recognise as sounding like the French for slippers—turns out to be Romanian for shoes.

False friends become a problem as you learn more of a language—

for instance the French word *officieux* surprisingly means unofficial—but to start with its much more important that in Romanian a 'bilet de tren' really is a railway ticket and that a 'medic' is a doctor.

Of course, not all languages are as accommodating as Romanian but all European languages have some similarities; even Finnish, which is a language in which it is perfectly possible to look at the menu and order the headwaiter, has the odd recognisable word.

Languages can be half the fun of travel in retirement but to begin with your problem could be simply to make yourself understood.

Communication

What degree of communication do you need? Well, communication can range from pointing at your mouth to indicate hunger to holding a philosophical discussion, but it's all a matter of getting over a message.

Basic

Imagine you are a foreigner who arrives in England unable to speak a word of English. What words and phrases would you need to know? 'Do you speak my language?' is a good start and could save you a lot of trouble.

If that doesn't work then, 'Excuse me—can you help me please?' is probably the most useful phrase in any language as it carries all the imperatives of an SOS at sea. It's a good phrase to start with but if you find it too difficult then try at least to learn the words for 'Please' and, of course, 'Thank you' and combine these with prepared phrase cards which you can point to.

Phrase Cards

I like the plain file cards which are just the right size for the pocket and avoid the impression that you are peddling dubious postcards! Select the phrases you need from an up-to-date phrase book—avoid anything that starts off with 'My postillion has been struck by lightning'—and write out the words clearly on the card in bold capitals. Phrase books themselves are usually too closely printed for the purpose and might be quite impossible for a short-sighted foreigner to read anyway.

'Please', you say, stopping your chosen victim like the Ancient Mariner, and then—having first established that he or she is neither a compatriot nor a linguist—take out your card and point to the appropriate words. Later of course you can read from the card yourself or learn the phrase.

If you are anything like us you could well get lost in a foreign city—

I even got lost in Benidorm once—so your first phrase card could be WHERE IS THE HOTEL SPLENDIDE? or WHERE IS SANTA MARIA STREET? or whatever.

Spare Cards
Keep a few blank cards in your pocket, together with a pencil, so that your helper can either draw or write down directions for you if necessary. Of course if the directions consist of arm waving and fingers held up to indicate, say, first left, second right, you can either trust your memory or write it down yourself. After that your next move should be to purchase a map of the area.

Keep It Simple
Keep everything to absolute basics and don't get caught up with the intricacies of grammar at this stage. Of course if you really want to, you could carry a card asking HOW DO YOU SEE THE ROLE OF YOUR FREEDOM LOVING DEMOCRACY IN A GEOPOLITI-CAL CONTEXT? but to begin with we are talking emergencies and WHERE IS THE NEAREST PUBLIC LOO? and WHERE CAN I GET AN INEXPENSIVE MEAL? should be about as sophisticated as you get.

Most people will be happy to point out or sketch the direction you should take—some will even take you there—but it's as well to learn the words for left, right and the numbers up to ten.

Sign Language
Nowadays the world is full of helpful signs, many of which are international, although silhouettes on some toilet doors can still be confusing, in which case the only answer is to watch the local traffic.

You should take time before you set out to find out what the most important written signs look like in block letters: DANGER being perhaps the most obvious and STOP. If you are going to Greece or Russia it's as well to learn the alphabet in capitals as this makes it possible to read many signs using international words like bar, restaurant and taxi, as well as perhaps helping you to recognise that the Russian for Chemist is very near the good old fashioned Apothecary. Learning the alphabet will also help you to read street names and so on which makes it much easier to get about.

Wherever you go, find out the words most likely to occur on signs from your phrase book. If you have a partner or friend with you write them out on cards and make a game out of identifying them. It's surprising how your confidence soars when you recognise a sign saying CINEMA or THEATRE or CARS ONLY and the rest of your party is looking about them in bewilderment. Introduce them to the game if they seem the sort of people who'd enjoy it—it could make a useful ice-breaker with strangers.

Phrase Books

At this point you may well feel that you would prefer to speak to people—if only a few words—rather than use makeshift communication methods. This is where the phrase book comes in, but it's a good idea to find a modern one and not to rely on your old school copy which was probably ancient when it was passed on to you. Phrases like SEE HERE, MY GOOD MAN and BE CAREFUL WITH MY HAT BOX are not going to be all that much help when all you want is to order a beer—politely.

There are some splendid phrase books about these days and it's much better to buy one of these as an introduction to the language than be put off by a heavy grammar book. One of the best for travellers in Europe, *European Phrasebook*, is published by the AA being a useful paperback in ten languages. It lists a tremendous number of useful words and phrases in English, French, German, Italian, Spanish, Portuguese, Dutch, Danish, Swedish and Serbo-Croat, and if at first it seems a bit daunting a closer inspection shows how many recognisable words crop up in all these languages—including Serbo-Croat where a sports centre is, would you believe, a 'sportski centar'.

It's great fun—especially if you have a smattering of one or two of the more common languages—to track down words like 'frizer' in Serbo-Croat (which is the same as *friseur* in French and means hairdresser) or to identify 'zwembad' in Dutch (a swimming bath) but, apart from helping us to overcome any fears of languages left over from schooldays, it won't get us very far unless we are among those fortunate people with total recall.

Marking Pens

Like most phrase books this one provides too much information for our immediate needs and certainly too much for most people to take in. Use it as a tool for making up your emergency cards or you could go through it with one of those useful yellow marking pens which make a thick line through which you can still see the print clearly.

These pens are terrific items for any informative books—providing of course that they belong to you—so be our guest with *Travel in Retirement* if anything strikes you as particularly useful.

With phrase books you could use the yellow pen to score through the headings of the language or languages you need for your trip. Try picking out the phrases in the General Expressions section that you are going to need often and mark them, together with their English equivalent. For instance, if you speak no French whatsoever you are much more likely to need—and be able to use immediately—a simple word like *bonjour* (hallo) than the phrase *Veuillez repetez s'il vous plait* (would you be so kind as to repeat that) which takes a bit of pronouncing anyway. In other words, it might be best to try the short and easy phrases first so that you don't get flustered and too shy to try them again.

It's also a good idea to mark the numbers up to ten—later you might learn to count up to a hundred so as to be able to bargain in the shops and markets but the prices are usually ticketed so your most useful phrase might be 'Too much', accompanied by a sad shake of the head.

Then turn to the Key Phrases section and again mark those phrases you will need most. 'Where is . . .?', for example, is liable to be more useful in the first instance than, 'Here is . . .', while 'How much is . . .?' could have more relevance to your own needs than 'Are dogs allowed?'

On an even more simple level, if you love apples but hate oranges it could make more sense at this stage to learn the word for apples and ignore the one for oranges. After all, you're doing this to increase your enjoyment and not to pass an examination.

Getting By

The great advantage of being retired is that you have the time to learn enough of the language of the country you are visiting to 'get by', even if you have no great linguistic ambitions. Molly's mother after the death of her husband Harry—the great non-verbal communicator—learned how to get by splendidly in French, Spanish and Italian.

Getting by will help you make the most of your trip and will almost certainly save you a bit of money; it involves picking up enough of the language to travel, shop, eat out and to carry on a conversation of sorts. Most people really love it when foreigners try to speak their language so don't worry about your accent; even the French are quite kind to absolute beginners although for some reason they take a poor view of those whose French is more fluent.

At this stage a book—and if possible its accompanying cassette— like *When In Spain*, the holiday maker's guide, published by the BBC could be a very good investment. It was written for a BBC programme but stands up very well on its own. We like it because it sticks to essentials with a section on words to learn 'before you go any further'—words like hallo, goodbye, please and thank you followed immediately by a useful chapter entitled 'Getting a Drink'.

Learning the Language

There's no clear dividing line between getting by and learning the language properly, but if you find it fun trying to communiate you may well wish to learn more and it's certainly worth it if you plan a long stay or frequent visits.

One indication that you are beginning to learn the language is when waiters and barmen start referring to tourists as 'them'—implying that you are a foreign visitor rather than a package tour unit. It's flattering of course but naturally the waiters and barmen realise this, so—like a yellow belt in the martial arts—it merely means that you may well be teachable.

Of course, when you are retired rather than at school the pleasant thing is that you are learning a language because you want to and the only person who can fail is the teacher. This could be a good time to join a language class, either in England or abroad if you are staying for some time in one place but ask around, study the brochures and make sure that it's the sort of class you want. For instance, if you have never had any formal language instruction you don't want a course which spends the first few lessons dealing with every single tense of the verb 'to have' and where the teacher uses words like Preterite and Past Historic which few of us understand in English.

It's best to explain exactly what you want to achieve; if you do want to try for an O or A level in French or Spanish that's fine but if you just want some basic holiday or travelling phrases then ask the teacher if the class is right for you. Local colleges often run afternoon or evening classes specifically for retired people. Molly's mother attended several for different languages but she also had a few lessons in pronunciation from a student. It's not necessary to speak a language perfectly—after all think how attractive most foreign accents are in English—but you do need a bit of tuition in pronunciation. Cassettes, radio and TV programmes are first-class in this respect because they encourage you to repeat simple, useful phrases and to check out the meaning in a phrase book. Above all, learning a language should be fun so, if you are not enjoying yourself and not learning the sort of things you want to learn—leave and find another class.

Once you've got a basic understanding of a language you'll be surprised at how quickly your vocabulary increases. If you are staying on a camping or caravan site, for example, you'll probably find people of different nationalities whose knowledge of the local language is as limited as yours but you'll both learn as you struggle to talk together

—and laugh together. Shopping at the local supermarket is a great help too as you soon learn the names of the various items. After a while you'll probably feel confident enough to go into the small shops and ask for what you want but in the first instance a self-service shop is a good introduction.

By this time you may be able to decipher newspaper headlines and some of the main stories, which are very helpful because there are usually one or two running topics which use the same vocabulary every day.

Television and radio are useful for much the same reasons—the news programmes are usually the easiest to get some idea of, and you can pick up the accent and the cadence by osmosis, even if you don't understand all that is said. Once you can follow even a little of the language, TV is particularly good, but don't worry if you can't understand the comedy programmes or the stand up comics—after all you probably don't get every word of a regional comic in English.

By now you should be saying a few words to the locals. Try not to be browbeaten by those who insist on speaking English all the time. Make sure you speak their language at least part of the time and if they show off their English too much you can always deflate them by lapsing into broad Geordie, Scouse or whatever. By all means agree to teach them the Bladon Races but only if they play fair and help you out with their language, allowing you to speak—however hesitantly— when it's your turn.

Learning languages when you are travelling in retirement can be a marvellously rewarding experience and you could soon find it impossible to remember the days when you walked around with your pockets filled with phrase cards. Not only that, but once you have become reasonably fluent in one foreign language it's as though you have broken down some sort of barrier—and this is especially true of older British people—which makes it a great deal easier to make yourself understood, to get by or to attain fluency in other languages. After all, even Chinese can't be all that hard to learn if hundreds of millions of Chinese babies can manage it.

Examples for Basic Phrase Cards

English	*Spanish*
I have a reservation	Tengo un reserva
On the ground floor	En el sotano
A return ticket please	Billete de ida y vuelta por favor
English	*French*
Where is the hotel?	Ou se trouve l'hotel?
Where is the toilet?	Ou est le WC?

Further Reading

Berlitz Travel Guides, Berlitz, London. Pocket-size books with phrase-book section. Lots of local history, maps, shopping guides, transport, hotels. Good value, and a useful addition to your standard phrasebook

Collins' Phrase Books, Collins, London. Hardback pocket-size series. A dozen or so languages covered over a wide range of phrases. Handy format

European Phrasebook, Automobile Association (for the Alliance Internationale de Tourisme), Basingstoke. Wide-ranging and covers 10 countries. But the print is a bit small and you may need to copy out useful phrases onto cards

France—A Cultural Guide, Phaidon Press, London. An A to Y illustrated digest from Abbéville to Yvoire with details of castles, musuems, theatres, etc. Excellent to pore over while planning a trip or to take with you in the car .

Get By in . . ., BBC Books, London. A beginner's course for the holidaymaker, published in several languages. Excellent value, simple style and covers most situations

The Traveller's Trivia Test—1001 Questions and Answers for the Sophisticated Traveller, George Blagowidow, Equation Press, London. Masses of off-beat information to catch out your fellow voyagers

13

Something for — Almost — Nothing

For most of us no longer in full-time employment money is something that has to be considered fairly carefully—which means that when we travel we are looking for bargains.

Of course, as we've already stressed, the mere fact of being retired puts a lot of travel bargains within our reach and we can save money simply by using transport at off-peak times and by travelling outside the high season when everyone else is on the move. This is fine and it does enable retired people to save a small fortune but it's only the beginning of the story for those who really want to economise. The fact is that just being retired is enough to make travel cheap but what we are looking for is cheaper, cheapest and where possible—free.

Cheaper, Cheapest and Free

You're not in a hurry so save money when travelling by taking a bus instead of a taxi, wherever feasible, especially from airports which are usually in the next county to wherever you want to be.

If you do have to take a taxi be prepared to haggle and if the rate seems over the odds check out the possibility of getting a mini-cab or the local equivalent. I was quoted £20 for a ten minute ride from Heathrow not long ago and actually climbed out of the taxi to find a minicab which took me to my hotel for £10—which was still extortionate but a good saving.

Save
By picking your hotel. The same night that I saved a tenner on the taxi I found that the company paying for my trip had booked me into a hotel where a mediocre room with no dinner and no breakfast cost nearly £100. Because they had booked me in earlier I was already listed on their computer which meant that even though the manager

was sympathetic to my request for a discount—in this case because I was doing some travel writing—he couldn't do anything about it.

Save

By asking for a discount. Ask for this when you book—*not* when you arrive—on the grounds that you are a pensioner, a journalist, a publican, or a member of the Royal and Ancient Order of Box Top Collectors. You may not always get a discount but there's always a good chance, especially out of season when competition is keen. Ask if they have a hotel car which meets trains or coaches—it's worth a try. Some small hotels in Britain even have private coaches which will collect you in your home town and deliver you straight to the hotel and for anyone a bit frail who has difficulty handling luggage these are well worth investigating.

Save

By avoiding more travelling. Especially if you are a man on your own, you can save by finding the nearest small hotel or guest house in the vicinity of a railway station; that is, one that looks clean and doesn't actually have a red light outside it. After all, if you are staying for only one or two nights at the most you are not going to worry about having a good address, a great view or a fine restaurant. Hal Newell in his travels all over the world has found accommodation by this method—among others—and he swears by it. He usually books in for one night only and shifts to another place if he's not satisfied. Even though he travels for several months at a time he tries to keep his luggage down to what he can carry easily and this is also a good saving as it enables him to travel by local bus, coach or train without too much difficulty.

Save

By abandoning snobbish consideration. Now you are retired you no longer have to worry about status. You have only yourself—or yourselves—to consider, so make a list of your minimum requirements anywhere you go. You'll be surprised how short it is because all you really need is somewhere central—which the older and cheaper hotels often are—with a room that is clean, reasonably comfortable and has acceptable toilet facilities either *en suite* or close by.

There are other advantages in using a cheap hotel rather than the ultra-modern expensive executive caravanserai. For one thing the rooms are often more spacious and the staff more obliging than in modern impersonal luxury hotels. Some time ago I was working for an American magazine in Monte Carlo and, although my expenses were open ended, I objected to the fact that at the first hotel I tried, as there were no rooms available, they wanted me to take a suite at

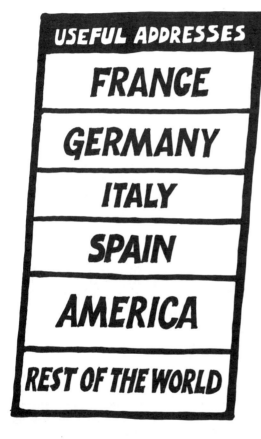

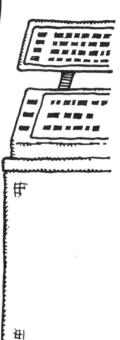

A few addresses can come in handy.

a price which I thought was incredibly high. Instead, after a hurried consultation with the taxi driver—always worth the fare on a short trip as an invaluable source of local knowledge—I was taken to a super old hotel in the middle of town where the room cost me one tenth of what the modern hotel had asked. As an added bonus, the place turned out to be the headquarters of the canny French press corps who were covering the same story and, as they were not in competition, proved very helpful indeed.

As well as helping save money on the bill you'll usually meet the locals if you stay at a smaller hotel and this too can save you money.

Save

By chatting up the concierge. In an older hotel the head porter will often have more time to talk to you than his colleagues in the 'palaces'. Like them he won't be averse to making a bob or two from the owners of local restaurants and so on by recommending their establishments but he's much more likely to have the addresses of reasonably priced eating places on file.

In a smaller hotel, too, the concierge will know you by name after the first meeting and will probably be a lifelong friend after the second.

Save

By being nice to the concierge and the rest of the staff. This may seem obvious but although hotel staff like money as much as the rest of us they also like appreciation. Give them both and you won't, as some people do, have to make up for your brusqueness by giving them large tips.

Save

By tipping thoughtfully, Molly's father, when staying in hotels, always tipped the restaurant staff on the first day, with a strong hint that there would be more to come if all was to his satisfaction. In total he only tipped as much as most guests but he got excellent service and a friendly smile from the staff.

Save

By thinking in terms of boarding houses, guest houses and so on. There seems to be some sort of rule these days that executives have to stay at flashy expensive hotels. No such rule exists for retired people and we can therefore check on the alternatives which are usually available at around a tenth of the price. Check out if an evening meal is included in the price—often these are excellent value—and, if not, ask whether there is a reasonably priced restaurant nearby. You don't want to have to walk miles in the pouring rain to get a bite to eat. Of course if you know in advance you could manage with a picnic for a few days but for anything longer you'd be advised to find somewhere more convenient.

Of course if you can afford a four- or five-star hotel where a bedroom could set you back more than £100 a night for the room alone, there's no reason on earth why you shouldn't treat yourself, but bed and breakfast in a guest house or private hotel for £10 or £15 looks good, especially as it leaves more to spend on food and enjoying yourself. These days you can still get a decent pub lunch in Britain for under £1.75 in the provinces. So, even if you go out for a restaurant meal in the evening you are still making a considerable saving by comparison with a stay at a luxury hotel. The same applies in most places on the Continent where it's always best when on a tight budget to stick to the fixed price menus. These are usually excellent value with no unpleasant surprises when you get the bill.

If you are staying in a large hotel, bear in mind that little things like drinks in the bar or sandwiches brought to your room add mightily to your hotel bill compared with a pint of bitter and a ploughman's in a pub.

Save

By trying Youth Hostels. As we've already mentioned, in the eyes of the YHA you are still flatteringly youthful, whatever your age and in most cases you don't even have to be a member to use the facilities, but the rates are generally cheaper if you are.

Save

By consulting the younger British travellers you come across on your journeys because, by and large, it's the youngsters who know all the tips. The generation gap is almost non-existent among travellers and young people are a tremendous source of local knowledge which they are usually glad to share. They know the cheap places to stay, the easiest and cheapest ways of getting around and so on, but there is one snag. The sort of thing an 18-year-old might regard as tolerable comfort might be sheer agony for bones 40 years older. It pays to check with them about hostels too as there is the occasional exception to the general rule about them being cheaper than the hotels. For example, in Jerusalem recently a friend of ours was asked £40 a day at a hostel while the hotel across the street was charging £36.

Save

By asking the local tourist office about accommodation. This applies especially if you've only booked for a couple of nights and don't want to stay any longer in your present lodging. They are usually helpful and can often fix you up with what you want at the most reasonable price—especially out of season.

Save

By also asking the tourist office for any maps, brochures and details of local events. Fiestas, regattas, art shows and so on can generally be enjoyed for free and it's worth staying on a couple of days to watch something spectacular. After all, you now have the time to do this.

Save

By finding out what the local police are like. Not only money can be saved here, but also time and hassle. Find out what they like to be called—which is usually the equivalent of 'Sir!' I always find that a beaming smile and whatever the local expression is for 'Excuse me, M'sieu l'Agent, I wonder if you could help me' works wonders, but a student friend of ours who tried this in Paris during the 1968 riots was thumped with a baton. Perhaps maturity helps! Keeping calm and polite certainly does. *Never* shout or behave rudely to the police abroad, however annoyed you feel. It simply isn't worth it. Even if they don't arrest you they often have the power to inflict swingeing fines on you.

Save

By thinking very carefully about 'optional' excursions. Some seasoned travellers won't have anything to do with them because of the expense and of course they are not simply organised for fun. The travel reps, especially, make up their salaries by running tours and taking a rake-off from the bars, restaurants and shops they persuade the tourists to visit. Of course there's absolutely nothing wrong with this as long as you are aware of it and have reckoned up the expense beforehand, and it could be worthwhile paying to travel in comfort to somewhere you've always wanted to visit, with a guide to point out all the places of interest and direct you towards the best bars and shops.

I usually take any tours that are included as part of the package because they are free, except for a tip for the driver, and they give you a chance to decide whether any subsequent tours would be a rip-off. If there are no inclusive trips you might try a modestly priced one to see how the land lies but take the precaution of carrying a small picnic with you so that if you are guided to an expensive restaurant at lunchtime you can say politely that you don't feel like a large meal and you are going to have a look round. The main thing is not to book up for half a dozen tours on the first day before you find out what they are like. Besides, you might easily make friends with local residents or people on holiday with a car who offer to show you the sights—for free.

Save

By comparing the facilities of the place you are in with those available at home. Hal Newell for example felt that he had saved a lot when he decided not to sail or go skin diving in Greece because he could do those things at home. Personally I love to dive where I can see

144

amphorae, broken pillars and the like, as well as exotic fish, so I wouldn't have economised on that but the principle is valid and it's not a lot of use paying a lot to see a movie that you can see cheaper at home or catch for nothing on TV.

Save

By using your caravan if you have one. As we've shown, after the initial investment the savings are considerable, even when compared with boarding houses and guest houses.

Save in the Sun

One of the really big bonuses about travelling in retirement is that when winter comes you can travel to the sunshine and live in a warm climate for about the same amount of money it could cost you to freeze at home.

Frankly, although I was quite prepared to believe that there were some good long-stay holidays around, I thought that living in the sunshine on one's State Pension was just too good to be true. Not only that, but almost all of the cheap long stays on offer were in places like Benidorm which in summer certainly is my idea of absolute Hell. That was before I plucked up courage to try a Thomson Young At Heart Winter Break Holiday to—you guessed it—Benidorm.

Mind you, the weather conspired to make the point about this form of travel in retirement as the coach to Heathrow arrived at our local bus station two hours late bearing the cheerful news that a lorry had jack-knifed in the snow, closing the M4, but that our driver would try to get through on the country lanes. The driver, who deserved a medal, did get through, although at one stage we began sliding backwards over a long drop as he manouevred to avoid stranded vehicles. All this made it even more incredible to step out into the sunshine of Alicante a couple of hours later, for a pleasant drive along the coast, arriving in Benidorm just in time for a swim and a drink before lunch.

This sort of holiday caters for anyone over 55—which put me well into their age bracket—but the hotel wasn't completely filled with older people and the nice mix of ages included a complete Welsh rugby team along with their wives and girl friends. My room was clean and comfortable, though not luxurious, and there was a decent little bathroom *en suite*. In fact it was the sort of accommodation for which—with the addition of a colour television and perhaps newer furniture—you could expect to pay up to £100 a night in an English city. In Benidorm not much more than that would cover a full week including your flight and full board, not counting a host of extras like welcoming parties, daily tea and biscuits, video films, getting-to-know-the-area walks and so on.

No travellers in retirement worth their salt, however, are going to go for just a week when a long stay in a hotel can be had for around £500 for 70 nights, again with full board and all the trimmings. I found the hotel staff uniformly friendly and helpful as well as being specially attentive to the older and less active guests, while the food was well cooked and appetising if not particularly exciting. In fact, as one of the world's more demanding hotel guests, I had no complaints and I thought the hotels offered first-class value for money.

All the people I spoke to were enthusiastic. Pensioner Ena Edwards, from Oldham, told me: 'The food is smashing. I'm definitely coming again.' A retired milkman, 77-year-old Albert Lomas from Clevely near Blackpool, who has a £3 pension on top of his State pension pointed out that his month in Benidorm included: 'Insurance, airport charges—the lot.' A 64-year-old widow and retired textile worker from Lancashire, Elsie Hirst, was there with a widowed friend for the month. 'It's really fantastic,' she told me 'when you add up what you are saving on heating.'

My biggest surprise was to discover that in the off season Benidorm not only offers winter sunshine but is a first-class holiday resort with lots of good shops and restaurants to be enjoyed at leisure, with very few of the 'Kiss Me Quick' hat brigade around to spoil things. Unlike many popular summer resorts the 'Closed' signs do not go up in winter. As far as restaurants are concerned it seems that hundreds of chefs from all over the world have flocked to Benidorm to live in the sun and make their pile in the summer but, surprisingly, most of them are still around in the winter, serving splendid meals for around half the price you would pay at home.

In other words, off season there is an alternative Benidorm for anyone with just a few pounds to spare after paying for their basic accommodation and it includes a long coastline to explore and a whole moonscape 'back country', with picturesque villages which can be reached only by local jeeps.

As we know from our long stay in the South of France, winter is the time when the real cultural life of the region blooms, which means that even if, like me, you are not all that cultured there is usually a *vernissage* (artist's preview party) to attend or some local concert or musical recital to listen to.

Local Newspapers

The place to find out what's going on is the local English-language newspaper—you'll find them in most places where there's a group of British residents—or, if you've studied the language you'll probably find the 'Forthcoming Attractions' of the local paper is one of the easiest parts to read.

If you are staying for several weeks you are almost bound to meet residents of different nationalities who will be keen to tell you about places and events of interest. This makes a long stay in an apartment—like the one Thomsons were offering in Benidorm at about £130 for 70 nights, leaving in November—look incredibly attractive. You have to bear in mind that this is for four people sharing an apartment and there is a per night supplement if three share and an extra supplement if there are only two of you, but you do get quite a lot for your money. In addition to the flight you get a well-furnished apartment with kitchen containing fridge, cooker, water heater and so on, plus a sitting room, double bedroom and bathroom. Food in the supermarkets looked good and was cheaper than in Britain while wine, beer and spirits were a lot cheaper. Bed linen is changed once a week when a maid, included in the price, comes in to tidy up.

Of course, some bills roll in inevitably at home while you are away but, as everyone we met pointed out, there are no ferocious heating bills. My maths isn't brilliant but I made it under £50 for two people per week for the apartment—which isn't bad for a place with its own pool and a snack bar on the premises.

Working out Basics

You have to figure out your basic expenses in Britain—maybe put your car up on blocks to save tax and insurance; it would help a little towards your rates while you are away. Gas and electricity will be reduced to 'standing charges' only for the period and, apart from telephone rental charges, there should just be your food bills while you are away. These may actually cost less than at home because fruit and salads will probably play a larger part in your diet and you can try out the local fish and wine at much lower prices than in Britain.

You don't really need to leave your base too often—even in an apartment you are entitled to join in all the activities of the tour package held at their hotels—but you could budget, if possible, for some regional exploration by local bus or train, and the occasional meal out, as well as perhaps a little entertaining of people you've met.

In Benidorm I met several couples who told me they were living very well on just their State pensions but even with four sharing this would leave very little for extras unless you had managed to save a bit during the rest of the year. Of course it's still a lot better than freezing through a bitter English winter but for those with just a few pounds more than the basic pension there is a wider choice. Like many people these days we have a miniscule private pension—no firm's large pensions for freelances—which makes winters abroad a very tempting option. Look for bargains offered by companies such as Thomsons Young At Heart—okay, try to find a name for an organisation catering for the over 55s. These offer long stays on the Costa del Sol, Majorca, Tenerife, Portugal, Malta and Tunisia (among the many companies offering special deals for the retired are Saga—a very useful organisation to join). Such companies also offer coach as well as air travel to the Costa Brava and pick-ups from local departure points at no extra cost. Travelling by coach saves you quite a bit on the cost of your stay as against travelling by air and if you organise a holiday for 20 people you can often actually get your own holiday free, with cash discounts for organising smaller groups.

Take Time
Take time and have fun checking all the brochures, talk to people who have been to the place you fancy travelling to and then work out the total costs, not forgetting any supplements and your ongoing expenses at home. If there is anything about the stay that you are not sure about, ask your travel agent or the company concerned to clarify things for you but be specific about your queries—write them down and don't worry if there are several points you want to cover. When you have all the information, try to budget for just a little extra for mad money, presents and emergencies—after all you can always bring the money home with you!

Getting Things for Free
We've already mentioned checking out the local paper when you're abroad to see what free attractions are taking place and the possibility of getting a holiday free by organising for a group. For a single person it could well become an absorbing hobby to find out what is available in this line and how you can sort out a free holiday for yourself on a regular basis by taking on all the arrangements for a church or social group. You have the time to spare and will be putting it to some good use as well as keeping up with friends.

Britain for Free
In Britain there are an incredible number of freebies and the current edition of *Britain for Free* published by the AA lists nearly 1,000 places of interest which you can visit absolutely without charge. Not only are they free but there is occasionally a charming custom of allowing visitors to sip or taste the product in the case of, say, whisky or cheese or to buy products at factory prices.

There are also Museums, Craft Centres, Cathedrals, Coal Mines, Art Galleries, Gardens and Castles in the list. Weaving Sheds, Railway Centres, not to mention houses of the famous like Hogarth's House on the Great West Road are free, as are many pre-historic settlements, barrows and hill forts.

It's almost a travel hobby in itself trying to visit them all and while there do seem to be more free sites in Britain than elsewhere you will find some abroad and they are well worth the trouble. This is where your reconnaissance comes in — keep a notebook to jot down places of interest mentioned by friends, especially when they add 'It didn't cost us a penny to get in.'

Exchange Hospitality

You can make a saving and also meet people by exchanging hospitality. One of the first things a journalist learns is the importance of a contacts book but while mine was pretty good I simply wasn't thinking ahead when I was compiling it. As a result, while I could lay my hands on the 'phone number of quite a few politicians in places like Singapore I can't for the life of me remember the names of extraordinarily hospitable people who showed me round the city and offered to put me up any time I was on the island.

However, now I'm no longer working full-time, I have started a new contacts book which contains the addresses of people who, often in return for hospitality in Britain, have offered us a free night's stay and to that you can probably add others who have suggested drinks or a meal 'any time you are in the area'. After all, a visit to a town you haven't seen before or a short tour of Wales or Scotland is made special if you include making contact with friends or relatives if only for a short period.

It's probably best to start close to home and work outwards and this is what we did, beginning first with family members we had lost contact with, one of whom lives only twelve miles away and is good for pot luck lunch any time — as we are for him. Then there is a whole bunch of relatives scattered throughout the North of England and Scotland, not to mention the Isle of Man.

An American friend — Joe — brought the contact list to a fine art by keeping an up-to-date file in a shoe box. He had cards for everyone, filed under different countries, with the following information.

SPECIMEN CARD: Name, address, phone number.
Last contact — visit . . ./letter . . ./phone . . . date . . .
Information: 3 children (ages) one collects matchboxes. H. likes travel books.
Big House. Don't mind if you turn up without warning.

Joe travels round Europe for half the year in an old caravanette which he can park in anyone's drive or is happy to spend a couple of nights in the house if there is room for him. He always has some small appropriate gift for his hosts and offers similar hospitality in America during the months he is at home. He has only a small house but friends are welcome to stay. Joe is never unwelcome, partly because he is always hospitable and doesn't demand much from his friends and also because he moves on after a few days. When he is back home he takes the time to keep up his correspondence and his file.

It is amazing to realise just how many people you have lost touch with. You could find, as we did, that having renewed contact to the point of sending Christmas cards with a long note followed by one or two letters during the year, it is quite okay to telephone a few days before you are travelling to an area. An invitation to a meal or even to stay overnight to renew old acquaintance often follows. Of course the thing about this particular exercise is that you must make it clear from the start that people you visit are welcome to stay 'a couple of days' in your home whenever they are in your area. The 'couple of days' is important as both you and they need a let out if you find that you can't stand the sight of each other.

Hal Newell is an expert at finding free accommodation in this manner and the way he goes about it demonstrates how to spread one's bread on other people's territorial waters. He always phones in advance, never stays for longer than two or three days, no matter how sincerely pressed to do so, and invariably makes clear that his home in South Australia is always available to friends, complete with his services as a native guide whenever he's back home. However, since he realises that Oz is a long way away he sends friends one or two letters a year, usually filled with interesting clippings from his local newspaper. He also sends a bottle or two of wine at Christmas time and rarely arrives to stay anywhere without a bottle of duty free liquor—which of course he helps to drink—and usually takes his hosts out for a meal. I'm sure he doesn't worry unduly about the economics of it but, generous as he is, he comes out on the right side compared with even the most reasonable of hotels.

In between friends he stays at small guest houses, makes a point of asking advice from locals and spends time working out the most economical way of getting to his next port of call. He's always quite happy to adjust to moving on a day earlier or a day later if a travel bargain comes up and this flexibility and freedom is something to take advantage of in retirement.

Many years ago when we lived on the Riviera we were inordinately popular—or at least our house was—and travellers from all over the world would descend on us for a free kip—some bearing gifts, some not. Most of them were unknown to us personally but had met my sister in New Zealand or had an auntie who had gone to school with

Molly's mother and all of them offered to put us up if we were ever in their area. Unfortunately, not having the sense we were born with, we neglected in most cases to put their names and addresses in our contacts book and missed out on free accommodation all over the place. Now we've learned the error of our ways and visitors' details go straight into our book.

Contacts

Contacts make all the difference to travellers and you may well have contacts you don't even know about. For example, if you are a retired dentist there is probably an association of retired dentists in the town you propose to visit or at least someone who can put you in touch with a retired dentist of your own age for a drink and a chat. He might then introduce you to a couple of other people. Journalists are fortunate in having ready-made acquaintances in virtually every country in the world and often the same thing applies to other trades and professions.

Organisations like the Buffaloes and the Masons, of course, could be useful but if you are a Mason do make inquiries from your own lodge rather than trying to meet up with foreign Masons direct because they are not always the same sort of organisation as over here.

The Church too, whatever your destination, can often be a good means of making new friends wherever you go—Molly's mother and aunt found this in Spain—and if you feel shy there is often an English church to help you meet people. Membership of Rotary makes you a welcome guest at Rotary luncheons all over the world, which can be a very pleasant interlude in a foreign trip and may lead to friendships you would otherwise not have made.

I met Hal in the street in Monte Carlo as I was on my way to book in at the Hotel de Paris—when my American magazine employer was paying for my stay. He spotted my American airline bag and shouted across the road to ask if I knew a cheap hotel—which, as a former resident of the Riviera I thought was amusing. However I told him the one place to ask was Rosie's bar, halfway up the hill, where most of the English-speaking yacht skippers foregather and—would you believe it—Rosie not only knew of a cheap hotel but was a friend of the owner and fixed Hal up with accommodation.

Over a drink Hal told me that his father had enjoyed a great success in Australia with the song 'The Man Who Broke the Bank at Monte Carlo' so I phoned the Press Officer of Monaco, a super lady, who immediately invited Hal and me to be her guests at—among other things—an official reception for some international TV producers.

When you are on the move all contacts are worth exploring and as a retired person you have the time to make the most of them.

Places are interesting but it is human contacts that make travelling fun, which is why people like Hal hate package tours and excursions which they feel isolate them from the people of the country they are visiting. On the other hand, you could find some very congenial travelling companions on a package tour and if you are a solo traveller you might find it much more convenient to be a member of a group when visiting cafes, restaurants and the night-life of a new place.

. . . and Free

Packages can be great if, as mentioned earlier, you help make up the package. As a retired person with some organising skill, a few friends and time on your hands you can achieve the ultimate in cheap travel by getting yourself a trip absolutely free. It helps of course if you are a member of a club or organisation in your area because what you need to do is to find enough people to make up a party—and you go free.

Sometimes the magic number is 10, sometimes 12 or 20. It's usually easiest to organise this sort of thing in connection with special interest trips like walking tours, birdwatching, historic garden tours and the like and many of the smaller tourist agencies will be pleased to make this arrangement—some of them even advertise the fact. Even some of the larger travel agents will be happy to negotiate, if not a completely free trip, at least a sizeable discount for party organisers, so if you are making arrangements for a few friends it's always worth asking.

Remember to *save* wherever you can by conquering any reluctance you may feel to ask about retired people's reductions, discounts, special offers and so on. They can only say no and if they do say yes you stand to save, well, perhaps enough for another trip!

Useful Addresses

Global Holidays, 26 Elmfield Road, Bromley BR1 1LR. Long winter breaks for the person over 50 years of age. Ask for the Golden Circle brochure

Holiday Fellowship, 142 Great North Way, London NW4 1EG. Telephone (01) 203 3381. An extensive range of special interest holidays

Home Interchange, 8 Hillside, Farningham, DA4 0DD. Telephone (0322) 864527. Information on home exchange for holidays. A fee is charged for home listing

Intasun Holidays, Intasun House, Cromwell Avenue, Bromley BR2 9AQ. Telephone (01) 290 0511. An excellent range of winter long-stay holidays and breaks for the over-50s. Ask for the Golden Days brochure

Intervac International Home Exchange, c/o Hazel Nayar, 6 Siddals Lane, Allestree, Derby DE3 2DY. Telephone (0332) 558931. Information on various hospitality exchanges. A fee is charged for home listing

Saga Holidays, Bouverie House, Middleburg Square, Folkestone CT20 1AZ. Telephone (0303) 47000. Pioneers in providing holidays for the over-60s. They also publish an informative magazine and have a wide price range of package holidays, short breaks and long stays

Thomson Holidays, Greater London House, Hampstead Road, London NW1 7SD. Excellent value long-stay holidays offered in many countries. Ask your local travel agent for the Young At Heart brochure

Further Reading

Britain for Free, Automobile Association, Basingstoke. An invaluable list of museums, gardens, historic buildings and other places of interest where entrance is entirely free

Europe on 20 Dollars a Day, Arthur Frommer. Still useful and interesting though published some time ago and geared mainly to Americans visiting Europe. Obtainable from Roger Lascelles, 47 York Road, Brentford, Middlesex. This supplier useful, too, for many other offbeat travel books

14

The Trip of a Lifetime

Now that we have time to stand and stare — or for that matter to ride and stare — any journey, whether a stroll in the country or a voyage to the ends of the earth, could turn out to be the trip of a lifetime. By travelling in retirement we risk making new friends, seeing new marvels and enjoying fresh experiences, none of which is likely to happen to us if we are content to remain at home.

New places, new faces, new foods, new sights, new smells, new sounds are all just around the corner and now, perhaps for the first time, we have the leisure to enjoy them. Mind you, while we aristo-crats who are no longer in full-time employment have a lot more time to spare than those who are still working, most of us have less time to waste. In other words, putting things off for a few years may not be the best idea we've ever had and, if we have been saving up for a rainy day, now could be as good a time as any to fly off to the sun and leave the rain behind.

I like those signs you sometimes see on Recreational Vehicles (RVs) — the huge motorised caravans which thousands of elderly Americans drive to Florida and other sun spots each year — which read simply 'We Are Spending Our Children's Inheritance!' They almost certainly aren't doing anything of the sort but at least they have the right idea about enjoying themselves while they can, rather than thinking solely of others, even their nearest and dearest. Of course we aren't suggesting that you should sell up and spend everything you have on travel, leaving your family penniless, but what we are recom-mending is that some retired people ought to consider themselves for a change.

As for us, I've always had a healthily selfish approach to life — although Molly has a nasty streak of generosity which I do my best to curb — but we have tended to put off things like travel and holidays because we were too poor, too busy or just too damned idle. Writing books about retirement has made us rethink our priorities to some

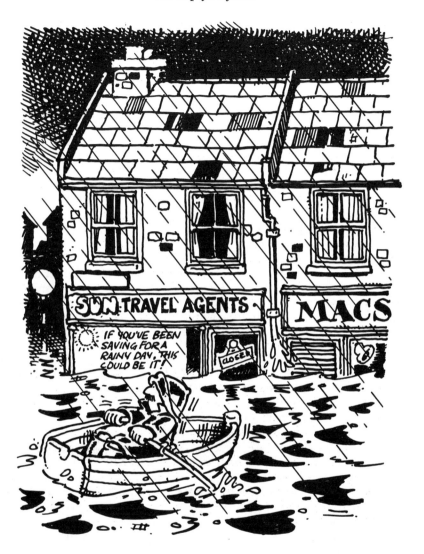

extent but what really pulled us up short was learning that Archie Macfarlane, the world's oldest sky-diver, had died at the age of 89 before the last couple of chapters of this book were finished. For a while we considered re-writing the chapter on rail travel in which Archie figures prominently, having used the railways among other things to go parachute jumping and mountain climbing. Then I remembered that Archie had told me how, in the battle for Beaumont Hamel in the First World War, he had taken part in an attack against

German machine guns, at the end of which he was the sole survivor out of the whole unit. 'Ever since then,' he told me, 'I've been afraid of nothing; I've enjoyed everything, especially travelling and every day has been a bonus.'

Archie had been retired for close on a quarter of a century when he died while walking on his favourite Welsh mountain and he had done his share of travelling. There was the travel to Hereford for the parachuting and to most of the mountains in Britain for the climbing—he was trying to climb them all—and then the trip to visit his son in Rhodesia. A little later, when his son advised him against a trip to South Africa, Archie used the money he had saved to pay for a flight to Iceland on Concorde and for a couple of local flights while he was there. More recently, much more recently in fact, he travelled by train to an airfield to enjoy a flight in an aerobatic aircraft—his prize in a British Rail 'Trip of a Lifetime' promotion for telling them that one of his dearest wishes was to go stunt flying.

Though he would almost certainly have rejected any such notion, Archie was something of an inspiration to the rest of us and for my part I wouldn't mind too much going out the way he did after 25 or 30 active and enjoyable years of travelling in retirement. The thing is that—partly because of Archie—we are determined to start our own travelling in retirement right now rather than wait for some day in the future, rainy or not.

Old Men Should Be Explorers

'Old men should be explorers', said T.S. Eliot, meaning perhaps that we older men—and of course women too—have the leisure, the experience and the patience to get the most out of new places and even familiar places. Certainly I don't think he envisaged hordes of geriatrics setting off for the Upper Reaches of the Amazon or creaking up Everest—though some older people may enjoy precisely that sort of thing. You don't in fact have to travel very far to become an explorer and any trip can be the trip of a lifetime.

If you have never flown in an aeroplane then a journey that some people might regard as a banal package tour flight to the Costa Brava might be the trip to remember, while for someone who has been housebound for years a day trip to the seaside or the country could be a big adventure.

In many ways it's easier for people who have not done a great deal of travelling to plan the trip of a lifetime than for the businessman who has retired after many years of international plane hopping. It's almost certainly going to be cheaper, because a trip of a lifetime involves pushing out one's horizons and if you've already been everywhere and

The Trip of a Lifetime

done everything this could be difficult. Don't worry though—it's not always a question of money or distance; some of the journeys I regard as having been trips of a lifetime have taken me only a few miles from home and a retired businessman could find his dream trip in a month's peaceful fishing out of reach of a 'phone.

A Trip to Remember

One trip to remember was driving a replica of the first steam locomotive, George Stephenson's Rocket, along Bristol Docks and another was travelling on the footplate of a steam engine from Newcastle to Crewe and being taught to fire the engine. Other trips have taken me further away—like the voyage to Icelandic waters in a Grimsby trawler, the one with the unfortunate luggage mix up.

Then there was the time a multi-millionaire acquaintance phoned to say he was going on a quick tour of Scandinavia in an executive jet he was thinking of buying and invited me to go along—and my trip to the Far East for a magazine which included a flight to Bahrain on Concorde.

The fact is that when I stopped working as a full-time newspaperman I more or less decided that there was no way any trip I might take in retirement was going to compare with the journeys I'd already made. As a result, for a long time, we hardly went anywhere; why bother to go to the Riviera if you've lived in Monte Carlo and why pay to fly to the Pacific once you've lived in Palm Beach and motored down the miraculous highway from Miami to Key West?

Of course I was totally wrong; I've been to some interesting places alright but even when I was living there I'd always been working and often saw very little of the place. Now all that has changed and, although I still sometimes write about my trips, they are not usually related to news stories—which means that I have time to savour them. They are also, more often than not, the sort of trips that anyone with time to spare can do without spending all that much money—like driving a pony and trap through the lanes of Somerset or sailing through the air in a balloon.

There's something else that's completely new about the way Molly and I now think about trips of a lifetime. Until fairly recently most of our journeys had been made separately and, to tell the truth, I did most of the travelling while Molly stayed at home, usually taking our many visitors on guided tours of wherever we were living. Travel in retirement is changing all that because for the first time we have the chance to travel together, even if it's only for a drive to the country. Already we've travelled several thousand miles together by train, car

157

and coach and we're planning to do one of Molly's trips of a lifetime by walking at least part of her native Pennine Way.

More adventurously, we're also planning to follow in the footsteps of our friends Molly and David Jones, who since their early retirement some years ago have travelled literally to the ends of the earth. Molly and David are archetypal travellers in retirement who left their teaching jobs ten years ago and are still happily looking for their trip of a lifetime. David got a taste for foreign travel in the Royal Artillery when he went to South Africa, India, Persia, Egypt and North Africa and carried on travelling when he became a geography teacher and started taking school parties abroad.

'Our first trip after we retired,' he said, 'was to Thailand and it's still possibly the trip of our lifetime so far.' Their second big trip was to Russia which they found exciting and interesting but not quite so enjoyable as their other journeys, a fact which they tend to blame on the fact that they were travelling with a party of Americans, mainly women. Then came a visit to California and the American West, during which the friends they were staying with took them down into Mexico.

In 1984 they went to China—a trip which cost them £1,300 each for 'a marvellous 19 days' during which they spent virtually nothing extra, not even on food. They travelled by train from Peking to Shanghai and visited the Great Wall, as well as seeing the magnificent 'Terracotta Army' but what impressed them most was the friendliness of the people, especially the children who were fascinated by Molly's blonde hair. The next year they went to Hawaii, which they found expensive, and then on to California to stay with friends and in 1986 they were again staying with friends—this time in the Cameroons.

When we talked to them recently they had already travelled very cheaply for 14 days in Turkey, spending extra money only on lunches at about £1 a time. As David remarked, we were lucky to meet up with them because the next week they were off to Singapore and Bali.

When they are not visiting faraway countries, they are usually off to relatively near places like Italy, which they visit twice a year to see friends, or touring Britain in the tiny caravanette they also use for day-to-day transport and for showing their many visitors round the West Country.

Molly and David have made travel in retirement into very nearly a full-time occupation and it's remarkable how they've graduated over the years from orthodox package tours to trips which involve an extra fortnight or so, often with people they have met on their travels and to whom they offer reciprocal hospitality. Said Molly, 'You can reach a point where for a trip of a lifetime all you really need is the air fare.'

For Ted and Dorothy Rogerson, elderly friends of ours who had never flown before, the undoubted trip of a lifetime was a flight on

Concorde, especially as it was arranged by their son who worked on the aircraft. For Archie Macfarlane, too, a flight in Concorde was the high spot of his travels although he had to save hard to pay even the relatively low fare negotiated by the Concorde Club of Bath—an organisation which arranges fairly frequent charter flights at minimum cost.

A Concorde flight is certainly a contender for anyone's trip of a lifetime and is an unforgettable experience as I found. For me the VIP treatment began in the Concorde Lounge where champagne and canapés were served. Then, minutes after take off, we were offered a Dom Perignon it would have been churlish to refuse, followed by a chilled vodka with our caviare as we flew twelve miles high, faster than a rifle bullet in a plane that was literally out of this world. Concorde is wonderful but it isn't cheap and while nothing compares with the super-sonic plane there are other flying experiences which are less costly. For dream-like almost silent travel, for example, there's nothing to beat a trip in a glider or a hot air balloon and although a balloon flight would cost you upwards of £30 it's not a lot to pay for a trip of a lifetime.

Many people save hard until their retirement or perhaps pick up a lump sum from their insurance company with the intention of embarking on their trip of a lifetime as soon as they've recovered from their leaving party; it's easy to see the attraction of a symbolic clean break with work or perhaps a super second honeymoon. Naturally your travel agent will welcome you with open arms if you tell him you have this sort of trip in mind but, although he can be of great help in making suggestions and taking care of the arrangements, this is one time when you'll want to see everything that's on offer, because sorting through the brochures and discussing the pros and cons of the journey is part of the fun, especially if you are planning to travel with a partner or friend.

Of course, a lot depends on how much money you have available but you shouldn't have to spend much more on your trip of a lifetime than you've been accustomed to spending on travel in the past—as you are now travelling in retirement and are able to take advantage of seasonal and other bargains. One way or another most of us will be able to afford at least one trip of a lifetime and if ever there was a time when we are justified in spoiling ourselves—it's now.

Certainly, whether you can scrape together enough for a weekend 'break' or find £100 for a Spanish package or cheerfully part with £60,000 for a luxury round the world cruise, there are plenty of interesting journeys on offer for the retired traveller who wants to become an 'explorer'.

Cruising, for example, is one thing that, unless you count a few short trips round the lochs and islands of Scotland, neither Molly nor

I have done much of up to now and a cruise could well be high on our trip of a lifetime list. I rather fancy the sort of thing offered by the up-market companies these days. Imagine being on board in the Mediterranean and the Aegean, which promises not only the usual luxury cruise but a guest lecturer to explain something of the art and culture and history of the places visited. I like the idea of the ship's restaurant serving the food and wine of the region. Certainly, a tour of Greece, Turkey, Cyprus, Israel and Egypt offered at 16 nights in an inclusive package including everything down to the tips, would suit us very nicely thank you.

On second thoughts perhaps a cruise on the *Nile Star*, again with guest lecturers, might be even more exciting; I like the sound of 'an informal cocktail party' at Heathrow to meet fellow passengers before taking off for Cairo.

One pleasing thing about travelling in retirement as opposed to travelling on business is that you have the time to make the sort of stopovers and side trips that were impossible when you were working to a deadline. You can play the tourist too, which means that if you have visited America on business and not managed to see places like Hollywood—now's your chance.

American Airplan, for example, have a Pacific Spectacular which takes in Los Angeles including visits to Universal Studios, Disneyland, Waikiki and San Francisco. I know people like Hal Newell think I'm a head case but although I enjoy travelling independently there are times when I appreciate being a tourist and when places like Fisherman's Wharf and Alcatraz are just my speed—and incidentally you can save more on fares if you avoid the high season.

Join a 'Down Under Club' and you qualify for flights to Australia and New Zealand at reduced return fares, with the chance to stopover in Hong Kong, Singapore, Hawaii, Bali or Fiji. This includes reduced price first-class rail travel from your local station to get your trip off to a good start.

Mind you, childish or not, one requirement of my trip of a lifetime is that it's going to have to be a conversation stopper and when someone asks 'Been away?' as a prelude to showing the snaps they took in Corfu, I rather fancy being able to reply 'Just got back from Venezuela, actually.'

Another thing I'd like to do is to take Molly to some of the places I've visited when working for newspapers and magazines, like Singapore, which I loved and where you can stay very economically for seven nights—flying Jetsave. A modern hotel might be pleasant but I'd like to take Molly for a meal at Raffles and also catch up on the trip I missed when I was told to 'stand by' for a job in Japan which I am still standing by for.

You have to keep your eyes and ears open if you are looking for a bargain trip of a lifetime because your local newspaper or local radio station may well have some good deals going and, more than anyone else, they can't afford for you not to have a splendid time. For instance, our local commercial radio station ran a trip to the Holy Land this year, which they actually billed as the 'Holiday of a Lifetime', as indeed it could well have been, including as it did not only biblical sites but places like Masada.

One advantage of this sort of travel, especially for older people, is that once you've paid your money everything is taken care of including coaches to the airport, excursions, insurance and all the service charges and gratuities so that you know all you have to find is the odd meal, a few drinks and presents. In other words you can budget for this sort of trip of a lifetime quite accurately and don't forget when you do your sums that if you'd stayed at home you would still have spent a few bob on food, heating and bus fares. When you deduct these from the price of a bargain holiday it begins to seem even more reasonable.

Another thing to look out for is the sort of long-haul trip, say to Jamaica, which offers a free third week if you book two. Three weeks at the Shaw Park Hotel for instance can be had for the usual price for two weeks. As a retired person you can take advantage of these where people with limited holidays have to rush back.

Of course, it could be a little while before Molly and I get around to doing any of the trips I've mentioned because if I can just lay my hands on £5,000 for the two of us we are going on one of the Great Journeys of the World. The difficulty—apart from finding the money—is going to be choosing which one we want from trips that start with a journey on the Istanbul Train from London and continue with offerings like 'In the tracks of Marco Polo', with names that roll off the tongue like Ankara, Bukhara and Samarkand, not to mention the rest. Just looking at the catalogue of these trips makes my mouth water but even allowing for 44 days for some of them I think we might find stays in some of the exotic places *en route* a little too brief.

One great thing about retirement is that you have time not only to send for and read the brochures but to make an in-depth study of the places you are going to—an interesting exercise and one that pays off all sorts of dividends, even at the relatively banal level of knowing in advance where the good restaurants are to be found. Wherever you decide on, your trip of a lifetime ought to be an adventure, and one I fancy is to America, taking the QEII one way and Concorde the other, which sounds tremendous and, as Cunard put it, is 'the ultimate in prestige travel, designed to pack as much enjoyment and interest into a few days as many people will experience in a lifetime.' Mind you Hal, who reckons he's overspending if he doesn't get a three month tour of Europe and his return flight to Australia for not much more than the cost of such a trip, would think it a fortune to pay for one day in New York — but then, he's just as likely to end up sleeping in someone's bath.

I suppose when you come right down to it there must be almost as many 'trips of a lifetime' as there are people who want to travel, as everyone of us has a different dream and the perfect destination is always just over the horizon. As for me, I'd love to take any of the trips we've mentioned and Molly and I are going to do our damndest to go on at least a couple of the exotic tours. But, if I had to choose only one, I think I'd pick a Round the World Air ticket, with as many stopovers and side trips as I could manage. The thing is, I'm still a bit jealous of my sister because while she has been all the way round the world, so far I've only been halfway before turning back — and it rankles.

Useful Addresses

American Airplan Holidays, Letchford Tours, Marlborough House, Churchfield Road, Walton-on-Thames KT12 2TJ. Special 'spectacular' holidays — Disneyland, film studios and so on

Hobby Holidays, c/o English Tourist Board, Admail 14, London SW1W 0YE

Ilkestone Co-op Travel Agency, (0602) 323546. Reasonably priced travel to exotic places

Jetsave Travel, Sussex House, London Road, East Grinstead RH19 1LD

Kuoni Great Journeys of the World, Kuoni House, Dorking RH5 4AZ. Marvellous, exotic brochure for places like Samarkand

P & O Down Under Club, 77 New Oxford Street, London WC1A 1PP

Princess Voyages, 77 New Oxford Street, London WC1A 1PP. Luxury cruises

Swan Hellenic Cruises, 77 New Oxford Street, London WC1A 1PP. Luxury cruises to the Mediterranean, Aegean, the Nile, etc.

Thomas Cook Escorted Holidays, 45 Berkeley Street, London W1A 1EB

Thomson Worldwide, from travel agents

Thomson Young At Heart, from travel agents

Further Reading

Australia — Beyond the Dreamtime, BBC Books, London. A beautifully illustrated history of Australia. Accompaniment to the TV series

Behind the Wall, Colin Thubron, Heinemann, London. A fascinating account of a journey through China

India in Luxury, Louise Nicholson, Century Hutchinson, London. A revised edition of the guide to seeing India in comfortable style

Japan, Peter Spry-Leverton and Peter Kornicki, Channel 4 Publications, London. A close look at everyday life in Japan from ancient to modern times

Maple Leaf Rag, Stephen Brook, Hamish Hamilton, London. Enthusiastic, readable, amusing account of travels across Canada

Samurai and Cherry Blossom, David Scott, Century Hutchinson, London. A journey from Okinawa to Tokyo which manages to take in history, philosophy, culture, food and the role of women as well as accommodation, transport and special tips for visitors

The Alternative Holiday Catalogue, Harriet Peacock, Pan Books, London

Touch the Happy Isles, Quentin Crewe, Michael Joseph, London. A splendid book on the individual islands, from Trinidad to Jamaica, by a writer who manages to conjure up the remarkable diversity and charm of each of them

15

Surviving Travel in Retirement

Playing the Old People's Card

If you travel in retirement—especially abroad, which most people do sometime or another—you will soon acquire special survival skills or rather hone those you already have. These are not a matter of health or security, which we have looked at earlier in this book, but more the psychological and social skills many older people employ instinctively and which those of us who are only just verging on the mature need still to cultivate.

The Good Old Days

For one thing, we have to learn to smile a lot and perhaps to say thank you a little more often than do the younger set, who can get away with taking everything for granted.

With hotel staff throughout the world, older people who play the age card correctly can establish an almost conspiratorial relationship, harking back almost without saying a word to the good old days when people knew how to appreciate real service. This often results in older people being accorded the sort of treatment in a tourist hotel normally reserved for patrons of, say, Browns or the Negresco.

Naturally, it goes without saying, we older folk should compensate for loss of hair, agility and so on by grabbing all the age-related freebies that are going—in the nicest possible way of course. Always ask if there are any reductions for older people and do haggle—pleasantly. After he retired my father-in-law became a superb haggler who never paid the full price for anything and whose magic words were 'And for cash?' Before he retired he would have been embarrassed even to mention money but older people simply are not embarrassable—or ought not to be.

164

Even in these days of sex equality little old ladies with a helpless air can get great hunks of men to carry their bags while pretty young things have to stagger on with their own. Men can often do the same thing but they may need a slight limp, which combined with oblique references to 'the war' can work wonders. Mind you, it helps to know something about at least one fairly recent conflict and to remember which leg has the limp.

One older people's card, which should be employed only as a last resort when charm and innocence have failed, is the irascible old person ploy. After all, now we are a little older we don't care all that much what other people think of us and a really good whinge accompanied by angry shouts, the odd curse and perhaps even a tear or two can work wonders—and besides, it's good for the system occasionally, so embarrass them before they can embarrass you!

A Country-by-Country Survival Guide

America

Attitude to older people Fine—after all, the British very nearly outnumber everyone else, but keep out of obvious no-go areas and, as a general rule, avoid talking about the Irish Problem in bars called 'Mick's'.

Language A minefield; the chap who said that America and Britain were 'two nations divided by a common language' was right, but don't worry, everyone will love your accent. This alone will be worth a drink anywhere (except Mick's) and will help you make real friends as well.

Food A pleasant surprise. American fast food is much like our fast food only better, but their breakfasts are splendid and, thanks to waves of immigrants from all over the world, their ethnic restaurants can be superb.

Austria

Attitude to older people The Austrians love all tourists, especially older people who visit ski-ing villages in the summer and you will be treated impeccably as the valued raw material of their national industry. The warmth is real but will remain impersonal unless you have an individual point of contact.

Language Austrians rather like it if you speak Hoch Deutsch or the standard German of Germany which they speak and understand

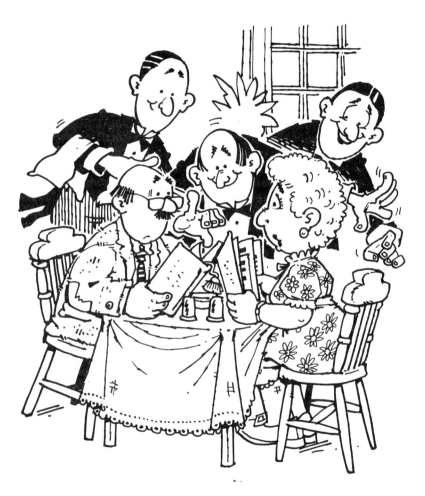

'Do you think we should tell them that the Duke of York we keep writing to is a pub?'

perfectly. Most of them will speak English as well, but among
themselves they speak a ferocious dialect which varies from village to
village. If you should understand the dialect, or even some of it, there
is innocent fun to be had by not bringing this to everyone's attention
immediately.

Food Terrific; if you have thoughts of diet prepare to shed them now. Everything is fried or served up with whipped cream or both. The chef who introduced me to the Austrian equivalent of *Cuisine Minceur* served me nine courses with appropriate wines and liqueurs.

France

Attitude to older people The French do not like foreigners of any age so as an anonymous *Rosbif* the best you can expect is tolerant disdain. However, they do love individual strangers and they adore eccentricity, so become an individual eccentric as quickly as possible.

Language Speak English unless your French is perfect and damn their efforts with faint compliments.

Food Splendid but only on rare occasions as good as they believe. Look for the *menus* to give a price guide and for local patrons to indicate value for money.

Germany

Attitude to older people Much the same as at home. Tourist welcome a fraction less warm but a fraction more genuine than in neighbouring Austria. It's okay to mention the war but, for heaven's sake, *don't* mention the time England won the World Cup.

Language Almost everyone speaks English with what appears to be a stage Kraut accent. They appreciate your efforts to speak German. In some parts of the North dialects are so similar to English that it's possible to carry on a simple conversation without speaking each others' language.

Food Goodish to very good, especially if you like sausages which come in all shapes and sizes and are excellent washed down with steins of beer. Some of the best restaurants are to be found near railway stations and underneath town halls.

Holland

Attitude to older people Super-friendly. Most Dutch people are very free and easy and have a great sense of humour—unless their local football team has had a bad run. Remember that the Dutch make a great fuss about their 50th birthday which shows their hearts are definitely in the right place when it comes to Senior Citizens.

Language Most Dutch people speak English so well it's almost a relief to hear them make a mistake. It's probably not worth struggling to learn much Dutch unless you intend staying for some time but they appreciate your being able to say things like 'Hello', 'Please', 'Thank you' and so on, and knowing a few words from the menu and how to order a drink is useful. You might also try to get your tongue round a couple of Dutch swear words if your teeth are up to it because even the most harmless ones sound fierce and the Dutch equivalent of 'Goddammit', for example, is guaranteed to get rid of any tension you may feel!

Food Terrific! We had a friend who used to travel to Holland once a month just to eat at an Indonesian Grote Rijstafel—literally large rice table—of 20 to 30 spicy dishes, served with rice—and who can blame him? Top-class restaurants tend to be expensive but provide value for money while lower down the scale there are plenty of places serving cheap hot pot, pea soup and so on which are a meal in themselves. There are also lots of Broodjeswinkels or sandwich corners selling soft buns with a choice of fillings, as well as kerbside stalls which you can safely use as money savers during the day before maybe tackling a banquet at night.

Italy

Attitude to older people Italians are extremely family minded and are therefore pre-disposed in favour of older people, especially as we are less likely than the youngsters to behave like rioting football fans when away from home. We are also less likely to forget that a church which is a tourist attraction is still a church and will usually behave and dress accordingly. However, older people are still regarded as fair game by bag snatchers and other opportunistic thieves so wear a shoulder bag like a seat belt, don't leave valuables next to an open window and don't flash your jewellery.

Language Many Italians speak English—most of them about half as well as they imagine they do. They will usually appreciate your attempts to speak their language and if they do laugh at your mistakes they will usually be laughing with you rather than at you.

Food Food is better for the retired traveller than for those who have to compete for meals, service and everything else with the tens of millions of tourist who flock to Italy at the height of the season. Make use of Italian friends—or failing them barmen and head porters—to

168

point you in the right direction and if the restaurant deserves a second visit find something you can praise sufficiently highly to make them remember you.

Spain

Attitude to older people The Spanish, generally, love older British people—if only because of the contrast with young British people. Just allow it to be thought that you hail from an older and more patrician era and you'll be fine.

Language Speak Spanish whenever you can, however badly. They'll admire you for trying and it's a perfect ice breaker, besides which, Spanish is an easy language for basic communication even though difficult to speak correctly.

Food In tourist Spain it's difficult to believe that the Spanish can cook anything except *paella* and *flan*—a sort of indifferent crème caramel— but follow the indigenous Spaniards for first-class cuisine or try some of their brilliant foreign restaurants.

Switzerland

Attitude to older people The Swiss are courteous and correct in their dealings with everyone, especially older people. Some of them can seem formal, even abrupt, but this varies from one linguistic area of the country to the other and in any case a couple of drinks usually works wonders. Most Swiss are far from mean but they do take money very seriously indeed and English-style self depreciation on the lines of . . . 'actually we're broke to the wide . . .' does not always go down well.

Language Most Swiss, apart from the country folk, are brilliant linguists. They have to be in order to communicate with their fellow countrymen as, in addition to Romansch—a Latin-derived language which has been an official language since 1938—many of them also speak French, German and Italian, not to mention Switzerdeutsch. A lot of them speak good English for commercial reasons and are pleased to practise.

Food Good and copious—especially if you like melted cheese which they use a lot. Cuisine varies according to which part of the country you are in but restaurants and hotel meals are often very pricey. Combat this by buying picnic food and a bottle of wine at lunch time and looking for a good restaurant for dinner.

Bon Voyage!

We shall be doing as much travelling in retirement as we possibly can, whether we are walking, cycling, motoring, caravanning, taking buses, coaches or taxis, seeking new destinations abroad by boat or plane.

We hope we shall meet up with a great many of you *en route*. So, no matter where your travel in retirement takes you—we wish you Good Luck and Bon Voyage!